The GAIT WORKBOOK

A Practical Guide to Clinical Gait Analysis

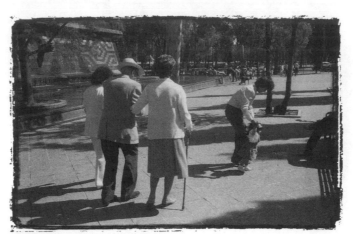
Photograph by Pedro Meyer

A Note About the Cover Art

"My mother would take him out everyday very punctually to walk, and he would fill his pockets with candies. He loved to give candies to the children. He enjoyed looking at children and I was amazed when I saw this scene of this child being helped to walk at the same time as the old man my father's being helped to walk. You are helped into life and helped out of life and all going on at the same time."

Quotation taken from CD-ROM entitled *I Photograph to Remember* by Pedro Meyer.

The GAIT WORKBOOK

A Practical Guide to Clinical Gait Analysis

Jan Bruckner, PhD, PT

Department of Physical Therapy
Northeastern University
Boston, Massachusetts

SLACK Incorporated, 6900 Grove Road, Thorofare, NJ 08086

Publisher: John H. Bond
Editorial Director: Amy E. Drummond
Creative Director: Linda Baker
Assistant Editor: Miriam Priest

A videotape, *People walking: Pathological patterns and normal changes over the life span,* complements this book. ISBN# 1-55642-350-0.

Printed in the United States of America
Published by: SLACK Incorporated
6900 Grove Road
Thorofare, NJ 08086-9447 USA
Telephone: 609-848-1000
Fax: 609-853-5991
World Wide Web: http://www.slackinc.com

Contact SLACK Incorporated for more information about other books in this field or about the availability of our books from distributors outside the United States.

Last digit is print number: 10 9 8 7 6 5 4 3 2 1

Dedication

I dedicate this book to my teachers, especially Margaret Mead and John Langdon, who encouraged me to wonder and explore; to my students, who challenge me to question and reflect; and to my husband, who walks beside me through all my journeys and adventures.

Table of Contents

Expanded Table of Contents

Acknowledgments

The work of Dr. Jacquelin Perry has motivated my interest in gait throughout my professional life. I deeply admire her scholarship and I acknowledge my intellectual debt to her work in the materials contained within these pages.

I thank my colleagues who read and commented on earlier versions of the chapters: Carol Ann Davidson, Ann Golub, Meredith Harris, and Beverly Jaeger. I appreciate their support and encouragement. Dr. So-Young Lee, a psychologist at Brandeis University, spent several hours with me enthusiastically describing her work on gait as a form of nonverbal communication. She then took the time to translate her findings from Korean into English so I could understand the results. Her time and kindness are greatly appreciated.

Michael Carasik typed the references, helped me locate sources, and provided bibliographic exegesis. I am also indebted to him for the reference on Akkadian gait that appears in Chapter 6. Finally, I thank my wonderful husband, Misha, whose love and support helped make this workbook possible. He is the quintessence of an azer k'negdo.

About the Author

Jan Bruckner, PhD, PT has a background in both physical therapy and anthropology. As a student of Margaret Mead, she began studying physical therapy as an applied form of anthropology. She wrote an ethnography of a physical therapy department and then decided to "go native" and earn a physical therapy degree. Dr. Bruckner has a basic entry-level Masters in physical therapy from Boston University's Sargent College, and an undergraduate degree in cultural anthropology from Barnard College, Columbia University. She earned a Masters and a PhD in physical anthropology from Indiana University. Her research examines the functional significance of morphological variation in the human subtalar joint and the effect of this variation on gait. She is currently on the faculty of the department of Physical Therapy at Northeastern University in Boston, Massachusetts.

Introduction

This workbook grew out of the materials I developed for my classes on human development and gait. The first five chapters and Chapter 7 draw on the scholarship of Dr. Jacquelin Perry and her book *Gait analysis: Normal and pathological function* (1992). I have adapted her work to fit into problem-based learning modules. I use these modules as laboratory activities to promote active learning by groups of students working together. Each of these chapters begins with a section on terminology to acquaint students with basic language and concepts. The next sections review basic anatomy, kinesiology, and the normal kinematics and kinetics. Activity sections and movement experiments help students better understand the concepts through experiential learning. In Chapters 2 through 5, the second half of each chapter is devoted to pathological function. These sections are followed by thought questions designed to stimulate thinking synthesize ideas, and enable clinical applications.

A unique feature in this workbook is the fact that students develop their own observational gait analysis forms. After years of trying different forms I finally accepted the fact that I could find no form that pleased everyone. I began letting the students develop their own forms. This process had a number of benefits. To develop a form you need to know the material very thoroughly, so this exercise required that the students learn the material in greater depth. The forms enable a high level of individualization. Each student's form reflects the way that he or she perceives information. It allows for individual differences and different learning styles. Students develop their forms section by section for the different regions of the body. Each chapter enables the students to add a new section to their forms until their forms are complete. At each stage of development the students test their designs by performing an observational gait analysis. This process lets students apply what they just learned while building on knowledge that they gained in previous sections. Their forms are revised and refined until they have a useful tool that they can take with them into the clinic. A companion videotape, *People walking: Pathological patterns and normal changes over the life span,* is available from SLACK Incorporated to help students with their observational gait analyses and the development of their gait forms.

Chapter 6 discusses variations in normal gait. It looks at the changes that occur in the gait pattern during normal development and the changes that are seen as part of the aging process. A section in the companion videotape enables students to see these changes over the life span. Men and women walk differently, so one section addresses this issue. Cultural factors also influence gait. Walking is not only a method for getting from point A to point B but it is also a form of nonverbal communication. Psychologists have shown that a person's gait pattern reveals his or her age, sex, and emotional state. These studies also have shown that observers make qualitative judgments about a person based on his or her gait pattern. Sexiness, desirability, power, and social status are some of the attributes that are communicated in the way a person walks. Cross-cultural studies show that gait patterns can also reflect a person's association with a particular ethnic group or society. Few textbooks on gait discuss these cultural factors. The demands of the clinic often mandate that a patient be discharged as soon as some level of independent ambulation is achieved. Clinicians, however, should know something about kinesics, the nonverbal language of movement and gesture, if they want to provide holistic care that truly meets the rehabilitation needs of their patients.

The final chapter provides clinical examples of gait deviations seen in specific patient populations. After addressing the body in regions and sections, this chapter has students look at the whole person and consider such factors as motor control, muscle tone, balance, and sensation. Students are encouraged to develop their own strategies for determining clinically what is a primary problem and what is a compensation. Understanding human gait and performing a satisfactory observational gait analysis are some of the most difficult tasks a clinician can perform.

This workbook was written to guide students in this process and to give them more clinical tools to help them improve the lives of the people entrusted to their care.

A note about numbering of the figures in the workbook: Figure 1-1A-1 stands for Chapter 1, Part 1, Section A, Figure 1.

Perry, J. (1992). *Gait analysis: Normal and pathological function.* Thorofare, NJ: SLACK Incorporated.

Chapter One

Basic Concepts of Normal Gait

Objectives

1. To define terms commonly used in observational gait analysis.
2. To describe the normal kinematics and kinetics of the gait cycle.
3. To describe and analyze normal gait determinants.
4. To demonstrate a fundamental understanding of gait deviations and their underlying causes.
5. To demonstrate some beginning skills of gait analysis.

Part 1. Terminology and Basic Concepts

Section A

Define the following terms in Figure 1-1A-1 and when appropriate give the average adult values in both metric and English measurements.

	Measurement Table	Metric	English
1.	Gait cycle		
2.	Stance phase		
3.	Swing phase		
4.	Single limb support		
5.	Double limb support		
6.	Stride length	70-82 cm	27.5 - 32.3"
7.	Step length	35-41 cm	14-16"
8.	Cadence		
9.	Walking velocity		
10.	Width of base of support (BOS)	5-10 cm	2-4"
11.	Angle of toe-out	5-18°	
12.	Head, arms, and trunk (HAT)		
13.	Ground reaction force vector (GRFV)		

Figure 1-1A-1.

14. Center of gravity (COG).
Indicate COG by drawing an "X"
in the appropriate place on Figure 1-1A-2.

15. Center of pressure (COP). Draw the line
of COP occuring in stance phase
on Figure 1-1A-3.

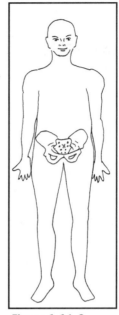

Figure 1-1A-2.

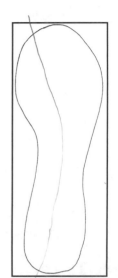

Figure 1-1A-3.

Section B

On Figures 1-1B-1 and 1-1B-2, identify the gait characteristics labeled by letters.

A. <u>Double limb support</u> B. <u>Single limb support</u>
C. <u>Angle of toe-out</u> D. <u>Width of BOS</u>
E. <u>Step length</u> F. <u>Stride length</u>

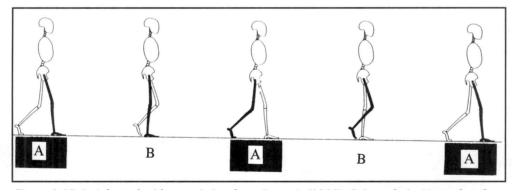

Figure 1-1B-1. Adapted with permission from Perry, J. (1992). Gait analysis: Normal and pathological function. *Thorofare, NJ: SLACK Incorporated.*

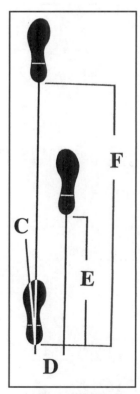

Figure 1-1B-2.

Section C

The Gait Cycle Terminology

1. Two sets of terminology are generally used to describe the gait cycle. Match the traditional terms on the left with the Rancho Los Amigos (RLA) terms on the right in Figure 1-1C-1.

Gait Cycle Terminology Table

Traditional Terms	RLA Terms
A. _8_ heel strike (HS)	_1._ midstance (MSt)
B. _6_ foot flat (FF)	_2._ terminal swing (TSw)
C. _1_ midstance (MSt)	_3._ preswing (PSw)
D. _7_ heel off (HO)	_4._ initial swing (ISw)
E. _3_ toe off (TO)	_5._ midswing (MSw)
F. _4_ acceleration (AC)	_6._ loading response (LR)
G. _5_ midswing (MSw)	_7._ terminal stance (TSt)
H. _2_ deceleration (DC)	_8._ initial contact (IC)

Figure 1-1C-1.

---

2. For Figures 1-1C-2 and 1-1C-3, fill in the appropriate subdivisions and percentages of the gait cycle for both the traditional and RLA sets of terminology. Put a star (*) next to the subdivisions that are periods of double limb support.

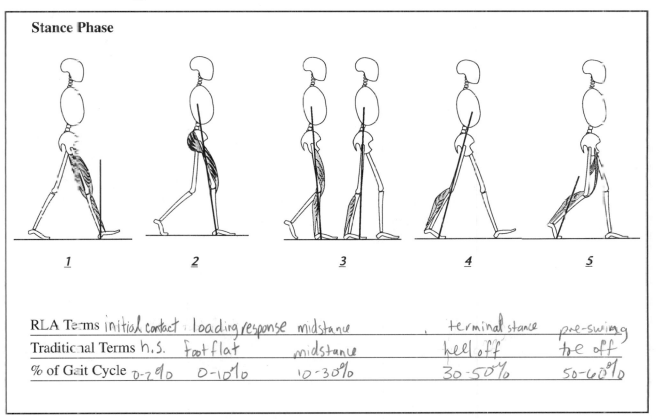

	1	2	3	4	5
Stance Phase					
RLA Terms	initial contact · loading response	midstance		terminal stance	pre-swing
Traditional Terms	h.s. foot flat		midstance	heel off	toe off
% of Gait Cycle	0-2% 0-10%	10-30%		30-50%	50-60%

Figure 1-1C-2. Reprinted with permission from Perry (1992).

Swing Phase

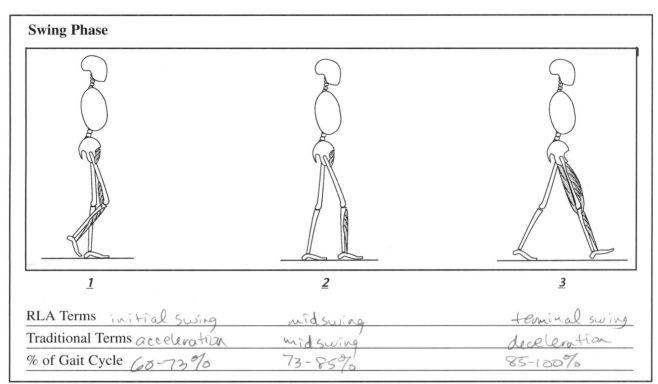

	_1_	_2_	_3_
RLA Terms	initial swing	midswing	terminal swing
Traditional Terms	acceleration	midswing	deceleration
% of Gait Cycle	60-73%	73-85%	85-100%

Figure 1-1C-3. Reprinted from Perry (1992).

Section D

Basic Functions

The Passenger Unit

1. Perry (1992) calls the head, neck, arms, and trunk the "passenger unit" because they do not directly contribute to the act of walking but go along for the ride. Elftman (1954) uses the acronym HAT (head, arms, and trunk) when referring to this part of the body. On Figure 1-1D-1, draw in the center of gravity for the HAT.

2. The passenger unit represents 70% of the body's weight. Discuss the implications for static posture and dynamic locomotion of having a top-heavy passenger unit sitting on top of a stilt-like locomotor unit.

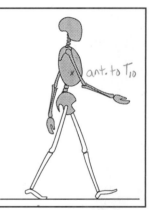

ant. to T_{10}

Figure 1-1D-1. Reprinted from Perry (1992).

The Locomotor Unit

3. Perry (1992) views the pelvis and both lower extremities as a functioning system that she calls the locomotor unit. On Figure 1-1D-2, label the (eleven) major joints of the locomotor unit.

4. Which body segment is part of both the passenger and the locomotor units? Color it in on Figure 1-1D-2. Explain the dual role of this body segment during gait.

   pelvic girdle - it is the base of the passenger unit.
   - " " " most superior component of the locomotor unit.

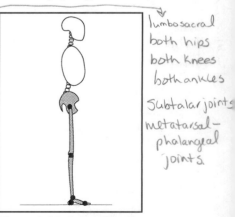

lumbosacral
both hips
both knees
both ankles
subtalar joints
metatarsal-phalangeal joints

Figure 1-1D-2. Reprinted from Perry (1992).

The Ground Reaction Force Vector

5. Recall the definition of GRFV. Under what conditions can this force promote a stable alignment? *GRFV promotes stable alignment when the COG is aligned over the BOS.*

   Under what conditions can this force cause torque at a given joint? *Torque is generated when the COG of the body part moves beyond the BOS.*

6. The GRFV is an imaginary line connecting which two points? *The body's COG and the COP on the stance foot.*

Quiet Standing

7. List three forces that control the motion of our joints. *Body weight, ligamentous tension, & muscle activity.*

8. List the close-packed positions of the hip, knee, and ankle joints. *hip-hyperextension; knee-extension; ankle-dorsiflexion*

9. In quiet standing, where is the GRFV in relation to the hip, knee, and ankle joints? *posterior to the hip, anterior to the knee; slightly anterior to the ankle*

10. Explain why muscle power at the hip and knee is not necessary during quiet standing. *both joints are in their close-pack positions.*

11. Explain why muscle power at the ankle is necessary during quiet standing. *the ankle is not in its close-pack position. The body tends to sway and muscle power is needed to control this.*

12. What is the normal amount of toe-out during quiet standing? *7°*

   Explain how toe-out can increase our stability. *- widens our BOS.*

Dynamic Stability

Contradictory

13. What is our width of BOS when we are standing? *3 in*

   When we are walking? *3 1/2 "*

14. Why is our width of BOS greater in quiet standing than during gait? *momentum + inertia help us out while we walk. We don't have them in quiet standing so BOS is wider.*

15. How much does our COG shift laterally during gait? *~1" each side; total 2"* Compare the width of BOS during walking with our lateral COG shift. Note that our COG is never directly over the stance foot during single limb support. *Avg walking BOS is 3".*

   What stops us from falling over? *muscle contractions, inertia, momentum.*

5

Normal Gait Kinematics and Kinetics

16. Complete Figure 1-1D-3 describing the kinematics and kinetics of stance phase.

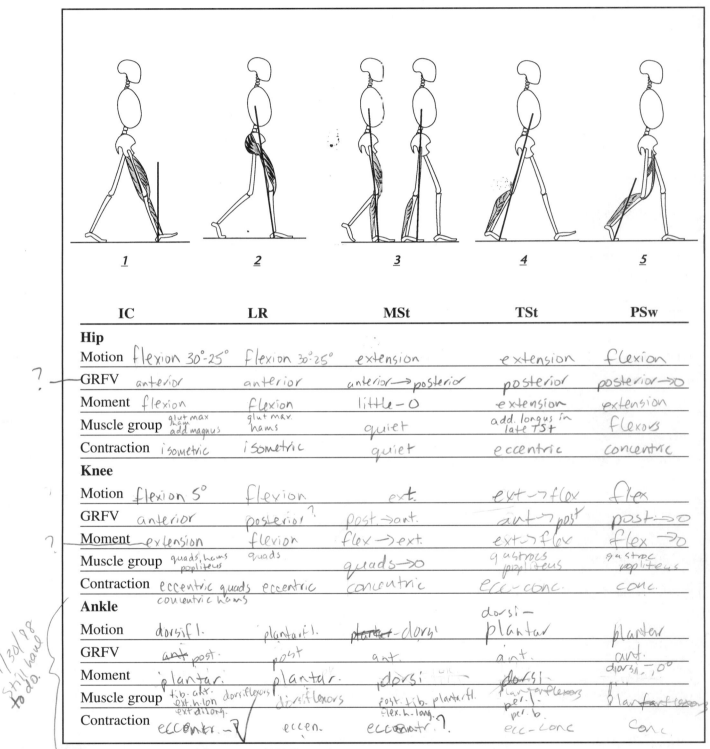

	IC	LR	MSt	TSt	PSw
Hip					
Motion	flexion 30°-25°	flexion 30°-25°	extension	extension	flexion
GRFV	anterior	anterior	anterior → posterior	posterior	posterior →0
Moment	flexion	flexion	little – 0	extension	extension
Muscle group	glut max, hams, add magnus	glut max. hams	quiet	add. longus in late TSt	flexors
Contraction	isometric	isometric	quiet	eccentric	concentric
Knee					
Motion	flexion 5°	flexion	ext.	ext → flex	flex
GRFV	anterior	posterior?	post. → ant.	ant → post	post →0
Moment	extension	flexion	flex → ext.	ext → flex	flex →0
Muscle group	quads, hams, popliteus	quads	quads →0	gastrocs, popliteus	gastroc popliteus
Contraction	eccentric quads, concentric hams	eccentric	concentric	ecc – conc.	conc.
Ankle					
Motion	dorsifl.	plantarfl.	plantar – dorsi	dorsi – plantar	plantar
GRFV	ant → post.	post	ant.	ant.	ant.
Moment	plantar.	plantar.	dorsi	dorsi	dorsi – 0°
Muscle group	tib. ant. ext. h. lon ext. ditory.	dorsiflexors dorsiflexors	post. tib. plantar fl. flex. h. long.	plantarflexors per. l. per. b.	plantarflexors
Contraction	eccentr. –	eccen.	eccentr.?	ecc – conc	conc.

Figure 1-1D-3. Reprinted from Perry (1992).

1/30/98
still have
to do.

17. Complete Figure 1-1D-4.

	1	2	3
	ISw	MSw	TSw
Hip			
Motion	flexion	flexion	flexion, ext. @ end
Muscle group	flexors	add longus gracilis	extensors
Contraction	conc.	conc.	eccentric
Knee			
Motion	flexion	flexion	ext → flex.
Muscle group	hams, sartorius, gracilis	hams	hams, quads popliteus
Contraction	concentric	eccentric	ecc → conc
Ankle			
Motion	pl → dorsiflex.	dorsi	dorsi
Muscle group	tib ant ext.h,ext.d.l →	" " "	" " "
Contraction	conc.	conc.	iso / con.

1/30/99 still have todo?

Figure 1-1D-4 Reprinted from Perry (1992).

Forward Progression

The basic objective of the locomotor unit is to move the passenger unit forward along the line of progression. To achieve this objective the body uses gravity as a propulsive force. The body is technically falling in a controlled fashion from one stance limb to the other. During stance, forward momentum is conserved in a serial fashion by rockers at the heel, ankle, and metatarsal heads. With the knee being held in extension, the whole limb progresses forward as the ankle muscles permit the foot and the shin to fall into gravity.

We can view the foot and ankle rockers as simple levers. The rocker is the fulcrum, the muscles generate the effort, and the GRFV contributes the resistance. For each of the rocker systems pictured in Figure 1-1D-5, draw a triangle in the appropriate place for the fulcrum, indicate the effort arm (EA), the resistance arm (RA), and the vector forces.

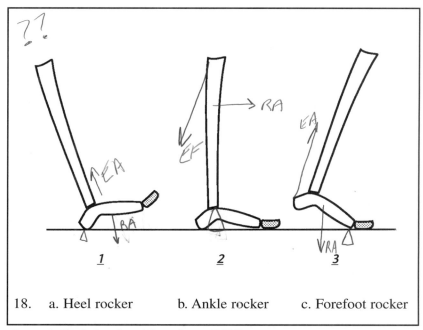

18.   a. Heel rocker   b. Ankle rocker   c. Forefoot rocker

Figure 1-1D-5. Reprinted from Perry (1992).

19. List four factors that maintain the forward momentum of the limb during preswing.

    a.

    b.

    c.

    d.

20. Explain how hip flexion during swing phase perpetuates forward momentum.

21. Describe the role that knee extension plays in conserving the forward momentum during late swing phase.

Shock Absorption

The body must accommodate the shock of impact each time weight is shifted from one limb to the other. Several mechanisms enable the body to absorb this shock and distribute the force over the entire stance limb. For each mechanism listed in questions 22 through 26, explain how it contributes to shock absorption from initial contact through loading response.

22. Ankle plantarflexion

23. Subtalar joint pronation

24. Knee flexion

25. Hip flexion

26. Hip abductors restraining a contralateral pelvic drop

Energy Conservation

To minimize the energy expenditure, the body controls its COG displacement and exercises selective muscle activation.

27. Vertical COG displacement

    a.   How much vertical COG displacement occurs during the gait cycle?

    b.   During which subdivision of the gait cycle is the COG the highest?

    c.   List as many factors as you can that prevent the COG from rising too high.

    d.   During which subdivision of the gait cycle is the COG the lowest?

    e.   List as many factors as you can that prevent the COG from falling too low.

28. Lateral displacement of COG

    a. How much lateral COG displacement occurs during the gait cycle?

    b. During which subdivision of the gait cycle is the COG most laterally displaced?

    c. List as many factors as you can that control the lateral displacement of COG.

29. Explain how selective activation of muscle groups minimizes energy expenditure.

Part 2. Activities

Station A
Gait Characteristics

Materials Needed

- *roll of paper (cut into 10-ft sections)*
- *measuring stick*
- *goniometer*
- *finger paint*
- *two chairs (for start and finish)*

Procedure

Use a 10-ft section of paper for a walking track. Place a chair at one end of the track and invite the subject to have a seat. Remove the subject's shoes and socks. The subject will paint the plantar surface of both feet with finger paint. Have the subject walk normally from one end of the paper track to the other. The subject may sit down and wash off the paint. Label the track with the subject's name. Repeat this procedure for as many subjects as you have.

Calculations

On each paper track, calculate step length, stride length, width of BOS, and angle of toe-out. For each variable, record the range of values (high and low) and calculate the mean in Figure 1-2A-1.

Gait Calculation Table							
	S1	S2	S3	S4	S5	Mean	Range
Step length							inches
Stride length							inches
Width of BOS							inches
Angle of toe-out							degrees
S = subject.							

Figure 1-2A-1.

Station B

Cadence and Velocity—Part 1

Materials Needed

- 25-ft walkway
- stopwatch
- calculators

Procedure

You need three people for each trial at this station: a walker, a timer, and a counter. The walker starts at the starting line with the counter. The timer stands at the finish line. When the counter says, "Go!" the walker walks from the start to the finish. The timer times this event. The counter counts the number of steps. Record the time and the step number for each walker. Repeat this procedure for as many people as time permits. For each person, calculate the cadence (steps/min) and the velocity (ft/sec). Calculate a mean cadence and velocity for the group in Figure 1-2B-1.

Cadence and Velocity Calculation Table—Part 1				
Walker	No. of Steps	Time to go 25 ft	Cadence (steps/min)	Velocity (ft/sec)
1				
2				
3				
4				
5				
Mean values				

Figure 1-2B-1.

Station C
Cadence and Velocity—Part 2

Materials Needed

- *25-ft walkway*
- *stopwatch*
- *metronome*
- *calculator*

Procedure

You need three people for each trial at this station: a walker, a timer, and a starter. The walker begins at the starting line with the starter. The timer stands at the finish line. The walker will be taking one step for each beat of the metronome. Start with a slow beat for walker 1 and increase the speed for each successive walker. Analyze as many walkers as time permits. Record your findings in Figure 1-2C-1.

	Cadence and Velocity Calculation Table—Part 2			
Walker	No. of Steps	Time to go 25 ft	Cadence (steps/min)	Velocity (ft/sec)
1				
2				
3				
4				
5				

Figure 1-2C-1.

Station D

Center of Gravity, Rate of Speed, and Variations in Gait Parameters

Procedure

Each person will do the following tasks while the other people observe the gait. Each person will have a turn being the walker until everyone in the group has had a turn. Note the differences in gait strategies between people. Walkers should take off their shoes. Put a marker on the walker's COG.

1. Take *very big* steps; then take *very small* steps.
2. Walk very fast; then walk very slow.
3. Walk with a very wide BOS.
4. Walk with a scissors gait (swing foot will cross midline over stance foot).

Questions

1. When the step lengths change, what happens to the COG and the velocity?
2. When the velocity changes, what happens to the step lengths?
3. When the BOS changes, what happens to the COG and the velocity?
4. Which gait patterns are the most tiring? Explain your answer.

Station E

Locomotion

Procedure

Have one member of your group *walk* approximately 20 ft. Observe the gait pattern from both the frontal and sagittal planes. Now have the person *run*. Each group member should have a turn demonstrating these new gait patterns as time permits.

1. How is running gait different from walking gait?

2. Describe what has changed in terms of gait parameters and subdivisions of the gait cycle.

3. Do the same analysis and description for *skipping, galloping*, and *running backward*.

4. Describe the gait parameters and subdivisions of the gait cycle for:
   a.   Walking

   b.   Running

   c.   Skipping

   d.   Galloping

   e.   Running backward

Station F

Abnormal Gait as a Function of Gait Determinants

Select a demonstrator from your group. The demonstrator will select one of the gait deviations below and demonstrate it in front of the group. The group will have to determine:
   1.   Which gait deviation is being demonstrated.
   2.   Which side of the body has the problem.
   3.   A clinically appropriate way to describe the demonstrated deviation.

Repeat this procedure until everyone in your group has taken a turn as demonstrator.

Gait Deviations

- excessive right (R) step length
- excessive left (L) step length
- shortened R step length
- shortened L step length
- excessive stride length
- shortened stride length
- excessively wide BOS by abducting the R lower extremity (LE)
- excessively wide BOS by abducting the LLE
- narrow BOS, increased angle of toe-out R
- increased angle of toe-out L
- decreased angle of toe-out R
- decreased angle of toe-out L
- increased cadence
- decreased cadence

Station G

Center of Gravity

Where is COG on an adult?

Place stickers on the COG of one of your group members so that the COG can be observed during gait in both the frontal and sagittal planes from all directions. Describe the gait as this "stickered" person demonstrates the following:

1. Little or no displacement of COG in the frontal plane.
2. Little or no displacement of COG in the sagittal plane.
3. Excessive vertical displacement of COG.
4. Excessive lateral displacement of COG.

Part 3. Thought Questions

1. How does pelvic rotation affect BOS and control of lateral COG displacement?

2. How do pelvic tilt, pelvic drop, and hip hiking relate to vertical COG displacement?

3. Explain how the following clinical problems would influence the COG and body alignment.

 a. A 25° bilateral (B) hip flexion contracture.

 b. A 25° L knee flexion contracture.

 c. A 30° R plantarflexion contracture.

    d.   A L knee braced in full extension.

    e.   "Poor" muscle strengths in L hip abductors.

    f.   A 25° R hip adductor contracture.

4. As the cadence increases, what happens to the other gait parameters?

5. What happens to your COG and your momentum if you have to walk at a speed significantly different from your normal walking velocity (i.e., either faster or slower)?

6. You give your patient a corset to help her low back pain. Will this support garment alter the gait characteristics?
   If you answered "no," why not?

   If you answered "yes," which gait characteristics will be changed and how?

7. Describe three sources of error in validity and three sources of error in reliability that may occur in an observational gait analysis.

8. Suggest three ways to minimize the sources of error in validity and three ways to minimize the sources of error in reliability in your gait analysis.

9. How does pelvic rotation increase the step length?

Chapter Two

Normal and Pathological Foot and Ankle Function

Objectives

1. To define foot and ankle terminology.
2. To describe and analyze normal function of the foot and ankle during gait.
3. To demonstrate an understanding of how the foot and ankle function during gait.
4. To discuss gait deviations of the foot and ankle and their underlying causes.

Part 1. Terminology

Section A
Functional Parts of the Foot

Define the following terms:

1. Hindfoot — calcaneus a talus

2. Rearfoot — " " "

3. Midfoot — 3 cuneiforms, cuboid, navicular

4. Forefoot — metatarsals a phalanges

5. Ray — metarsals + their associated cuneiform bones

6. Longitudinal arch — hindfoot, midfoot, metatarsals

Section B

Motions of the Foot and Ankle

Define the following terms:

1. Dorsiflexion – occurs in sagittal plane; around a frontal-transverse axis; distal foot approaches shin.

2. Plantarflexion – occurs in sagittal plane; around a frontal-transverse axis; distal foot moves away from shin.

3 motions} sup. add. altogether dorsi

3. Inversion – frontal plane around a sagittal-transverse axis; plantar aspect of foot moves toward midline of body

4. Eversion – " " " " " " " ; " " " away " " " " "

Single motion — 5. Adduction – transverse plane around sagittal-frontal axis; distal foot moves toward midline

single motion — 6. Abduction " " " " " " " " " away midline

7. Supination – triplanar motion of the foot around oblique axis combination of 3 motions: add., inv., plantarfl.

8. Pronation – " " " " " " " " " " " : abd., ev., dorsifl.

Section C

Deformities of the Foot and Ankle

Define the following terms:

1. Equinus – sagittal plane deformity; foot fixed in plantarflexion.

2. Calcaneovarus – ankle joint is fixed in dorsiflexion; foot fixed in inversion

3. Pes cavus – sagittal plane deformity; abnormally high longitudinal arch.

flat foot — 4. Pes planus " " " ; " low " ' also, feet fixed in pronation.

5. Talipes calcaneus – ankle fixed in dorsiflexion

6. Hindfoot varus – frontal plane deformity, calcaneus is deviated toward midline & plantar aspect of foot turned medially.

7. Hindfoot valgus – " " " " " " laterally away

8. Forefoot varus – metatarsals are deviated toward midline.
└Dominic demonstrated. No straight line between hindfoot & forefoot.
Subtalar joint in neutral
inversion of forefoot on hindfoot.

9. Forefoot valgus — " " " away midline.
 eversion of forefoot on hindfoot.

10. Hallux abductovalgus (HAV) — *a deformity involving all 3 planes; midfoot hyper-pronates, resulting in a collapse of the medial longitudinal arch & a medial rotation of the 1st ray. In this new position, the long flexor muscles of the hallux pull the big toe laterally when they contract.*

Part 2. Normal Functional Anatomy

Section A

Osteology

Label all the bones of the foot on Figures 2-2A-1 and 2-2A-2.

Indicate the location of the talocrural joint, the subtalar joint, and the transverse tarsal joints.

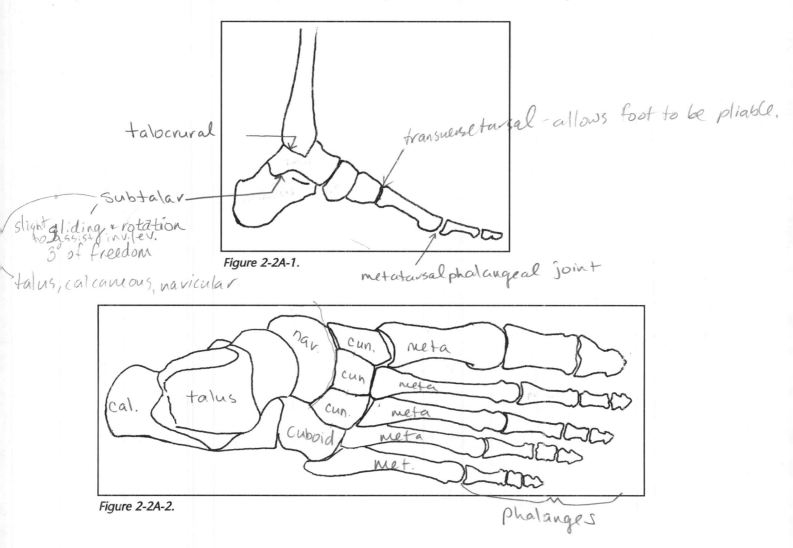

talocrural

transverse tarsal - allows foot to be pliable.

subtalar

slight gliding & rotation to assist inv.&ev.
3° of freedom
talus, calcaneous, navicular

metatarsal phalangeal joint

Figure 2-2A-1.

cal. *talus* *nav.* *cun.* *cun* *cun.* *cuboid* *meta* *meta* *meta* *meta* *met.*

phalanges

Figure 2-2A-2.

Section B
Arthrology

The Talocrural Joint

1. What motions occur at the talocrural joint? *dorsiflexion & plantarflexion*

   What is the orientation of the joint axis? *transverse*

2. What is the close-packed position of the talocrural joint? *dorsiflexion*

3. What is the capsular pattern of this joint? *more limitation of plantarflexion than dorsiflexion w/ a hard end-feel. If problem with foot, you would have a problem pointing toe not dorsiflexing it.*

4. In which position does the talocrural joint have the least amount of intra-articular pressure? *15° plantarflex.*

The Subtalar Joint

1. What motions occur at the subtalar joint? *Supination & pronation / inv./ev.*

2. What is the close-packed position of this joint? *Supination*

3. The articular surfaces of the subtalar joint exhibit a considerable amount of normal variation. Look at the illustrations (Figure 2-2B-1) of superior views of calcanei and inferior views of matching tali. Compare these illustrations with bones from your osteology lab. Select calcanei and matching tali for as many articular variations as you can find. Glide the tali over their matching calcanei. What are the implications of the variations in joint geometry for joint range of motion (ROM) and function?

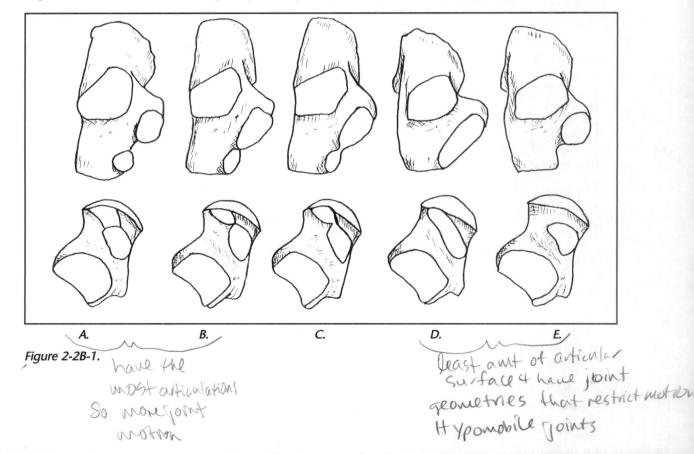

A.   B.   C.   D.   E.

Figure 2-2B-1.

have the most articulations so more joint motion

least amt of articular surface & have joint geometries that restrict motion Hypomobile joints

4. Inman and Mann (1973) depicted the subtalar joint as having a single, stationary oblique axis. They wrote that this axis caused the subtalar joint to function like a "mitered hinge" and they used this model to illustrate the relationship between internal and external rotation of the shin, and supination and pronation of the foot.

What is a mitered hinge?

Inman-Mann Subtalar Joint Model

Make your own model of the Inman-Mann mitered hinge joint. Fold a square piece of paper diagonally and cut a 1 inch strip off of a side adjacent to the right angle. When you open up this strip the paper should be shaped like an "L" and have a 45° fold between the two segments. Place the edge of one segment securely on a tabletop. Gently rotate the upright segment. Note what motion occurs to the segment on the tabletop.

pronate foot, medially rotate tibia

Supinate foot, external rotate tibia

In an open chain situation, what is the relationship between rotation of the shin and motion of the foot? Demonstrate these motions. *Foot supinated, shin ext. rot.; Foot pronated, shin int. rot.* *maybe not* *maybe not,*

In a closed chain situation, what is the relationship between rotation of the shin and motion of the foot? Demonstrate these motions.

5. Variations in the subtalar axis: Isman and Inman (1969) described considerable variation in the orientation of the subtalar joint axis. They calculated the average subtalar axis to be elevated 41° ± 9° from the horizontal plane (range: 20°-68°) and medially deviated 23° ± 11° from the midline of the foot (range: 4°-47°). Manter (1941) and Root, Weed, Sgarlato, and Bluth (1966) found similar results.

What are the implications of variations in subtalar axis orientation for foot function? (Hint: modify your paper model of Inman's mitered hinge so that the angle between the two segments is significantly greater or less than 45°. How does the change in the angle affect the movement of the segments?)
<45° more rotation of tibia because ∠ is more acute (sharper)(smaller in #). relationship between tibia & foot is stronger

Recent studies of subtalar joint kinematics challenge the idea that this joint has a single, stationary oblique axis. Engsberg (1987), Siegler, Chen, and Schneck (1988), Kirby (1989), and Baker, Bruckner, and Langdon (1992) described the joint as having a single moving axis or multiple axes of rotation.

Name another joint that has a moving axis of rotation. *Knee*

Describe how the moving axis affects joint function. *The femoral condyles glide & roll on the tibial plateau.*

What are the implications of a single moving axis or multiple axes of rotation for subtalar function?
More difficult to treat if dysfunction occurs,

Section C

The Arches of the Foot

The foot has three arches. List them and explain how they function during gait. Label them on Figures 2-2C-1, 2-2C-2, and 2-2C-3.

1.

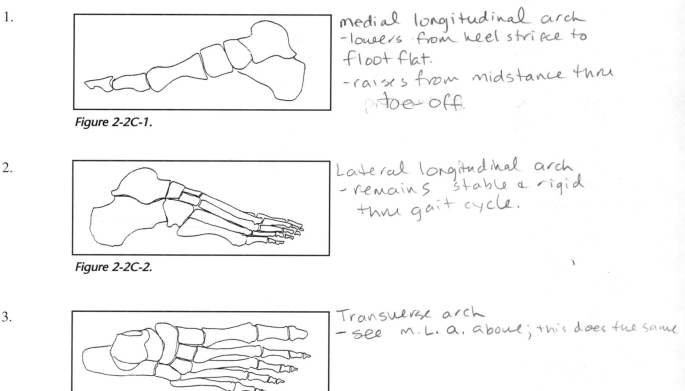

Figure 2-2C-1.

medial longitudinal arch
-lowers from heel strike to foot flat.
-raises from midstance thru toe-off.

2.

Figure 2-2C-2.

Lateral longitudinal arch
-remains stable & rigid thru gait cycle.

3.

Figure 2-2C-3.

Transverse arch
-see m.L.a. above; this does the same

4. What happens to the medial longitudinal arch when the foot pronates during stance? lowers

5. What happens to the medial longitudinal arch when the foot supinates during stance? rises

6. What happens to the lateral longitudinal arch during stance phase? remains stationery.

7. Describe how the ligaments and plantar aponeurosis support the longitudinal arches.

8. Explain how problems with the longitudinal arches can result in plantar fasciitis or calcaneal heel spurs.

9. Look at the diagrams in Figure 2-2C-4 and explain the action of the peroneal longus pulley. (Hint: What are the osseous attachments of peroneus longus?)

When is peroneus longus active during the gait cycle?

(Explain the action of this muscle during gait.)

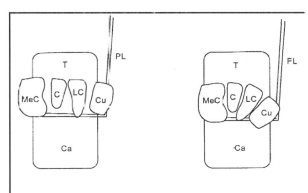

Figure 2-2C-4. Frontal view of midfoot: MeC = medial cuneiform, C = middle cuneiform, LC = lateral cuneiform, Cu = cuboid, FL = peroneous longus, T = talus, Ca = calcaneus.

Part 3. Normal Foot and Ankle Function—Sagittal Plane

Section A
Kinematics

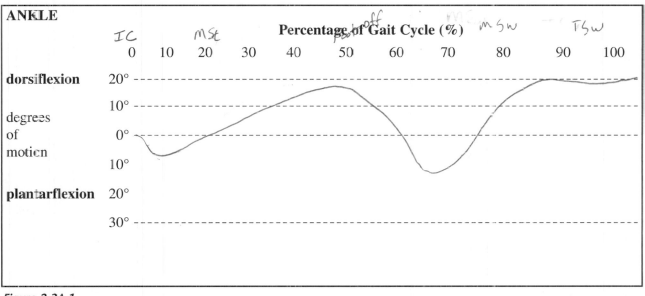

Figure 2-3A-1.

On Figure 2-3A-1 showing ankle ROM, draw in the curve that describes the movement of the ankle joint during the gait cycle.

Section B
Kinetics

On Figures 2-3B-1 and 2-3B-2, label each electromyogram (EMG) tracing with the name of the appropriate muscles. Gray areas indicate variations in muscle activation between subjects.

Muscle Name

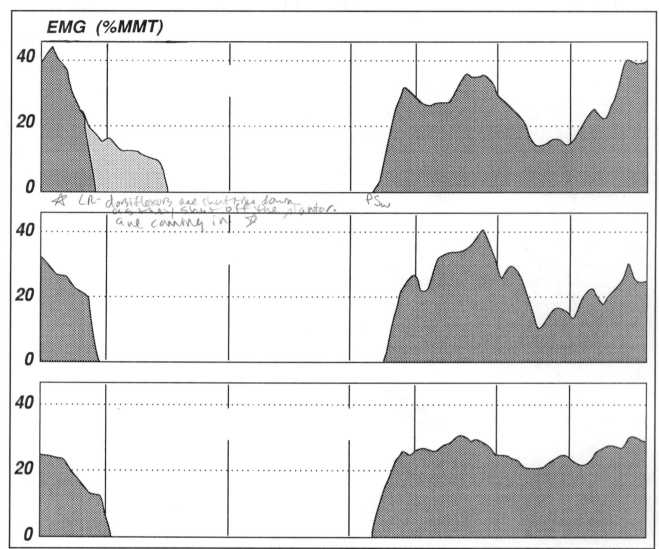

Figure 2-3B-1. EMG = electromyogram; MMT = manual muscle test. Reprinted from Perry (1992).

Muscle Name

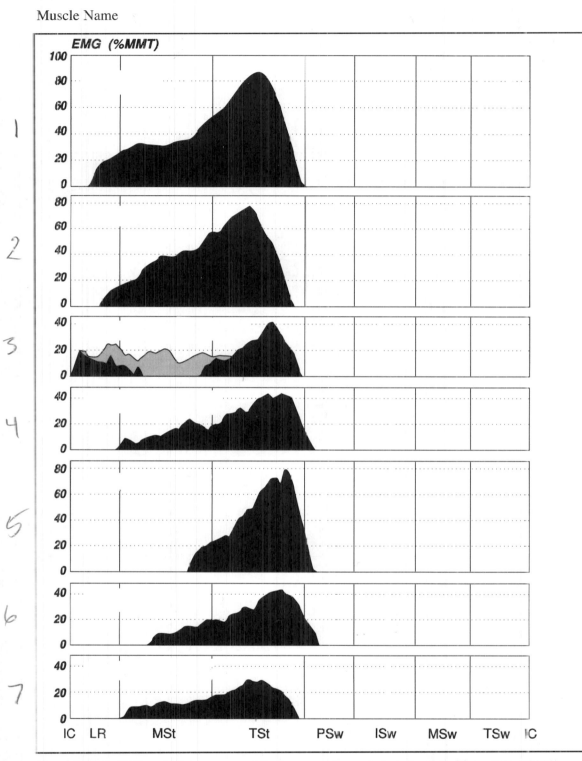

Figure 2-3B-2. EMG = electromyogram; MMT = manual muscle test. Reprinted from Perry (1992).

During which of the subdivision(s) of gait do the following occur (Figure 2-3B-3)?

Gait Subdivision Table
1.Maximal dorsiflexion (ROM)
2.Maximal plantarflexion (ROM)
3.Ankle dorsiflexor activity (MMT)
4.Ankle plantarflexor activity (MMT)

Handwritten annotations:
TSt – heel off
ISw – acceleration
foot flat   toe off   accel.   midswing   deceleration
– LR, PSw, ISw, MSw, TSw
midstance   – heel off
MSt, TSt

Figure 2-3B-3.

Explain the relationship between the position of the ankle (ROM) and the activation of specific muscle groups (EMG).

Part 4. Normal Foot and Ankle Function—Frontal Plane

Section A
Kinematics

On Figure 2-4A-1 showing subtalar ROM, draw in the curve that describes the movement of the subtalar joint during the gait cycle.

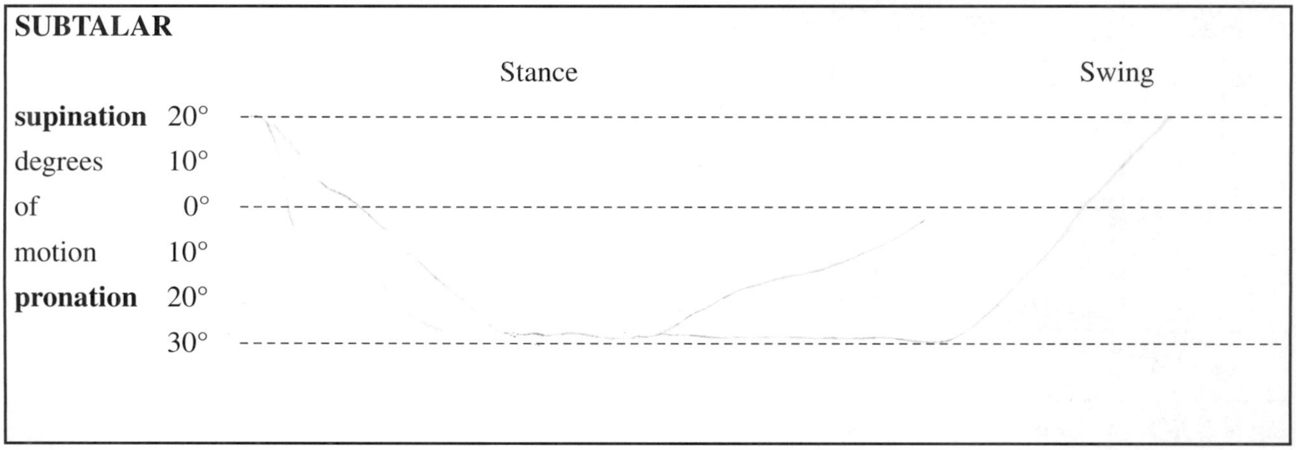

SUBTALAR

		Stance	Swing
supination	20°		
degrees	10°		
of	0°		
motion	10°		
pronation	20°		
	30°		

Figure 2-4A-1.

Section B

Kinetics

1. List all the muscles that pronate the foot and ankle.
   Peroneus longus, e.d.l., slight e.h.l.
   " brevis

2. List all the muscles that supinate the foot and ankle.
   Plantarflexor muscles, tibialis post., flexor hallucis longus, flexor digitorum longus,
   L gastroc & soleus   plantaris

3. When is the hindfoot in maximal pronation? Loading Response (foot flat)

4. When is the hindfoot in maximal supination? PSw (toe off)

5. Explain the relationship between the position of the foot and the activation of the muscles that supinate
   and pronate it. muscles are working eccentrically

sort of understand

Part 5. Pathomechanics of the Foot

Section A

Pathomechanics—Excessive Ankle Plantarflexion

1. On Figure 2-5A-1 showing ankle ROM, copy the curve that you drew in Figure 2-4A-1 describing the movement of the talocrural joint during the gait cycle. Place a star on the curve at initial contact (IC), midstance (MSt), terminal stance (TSt), midswing (MSw), and terminal swing (TSw). At these times during the gait cycle you will see gait deviations if your patient has excessive ankle plantarflexion.

ANKLE	Percentage of Gait Cycle (%)										
	0	10	20	30	40	50	60	70	80	90	100
dorsiflexion	20° --										
degrees	10°										
of	0°										
motion											
	10°										
plantarflexion	20°										
	30° --										

Figure 2-5A-1.

2. List three noncontractile reasons why a patient would exhibit excessive plantarflexion during the gait cycle. Briefly explain your answers. Include in your answers a discussion of when these gait deviations occur.

my own answers, look in back of book.

   a. Dorsiflexors (T.A., ext.d.l., ext.h.l) not working

   b. Longitudinal arch problem

   c. contracture

3. List two contractile reasons why a patient would exhibit excessive plantarflexion during the gait cycle. Briefly explain your answers. Include in your answers a discussion of when these gait deviations occur.

   a.

   b.

4. Perry (1992) explained that some patients demonstrate excessive plantarflexion as a strategy for protecting a weak quadriceps muscle. Explain how this strategy works. Include in your answer a discussion of when this gait deviation occurs and what other gait deviations usually accompany it.

Section B

Pathomechanics—Excessive Ankle Dorsiflexion

Excessive ankle dorsiflexion or the lack of normal plantarflexion can be seen in most of the subdivisions of the gait cycle.

1. Explain what Perry (1992) meant when she wrote, "Excessive dorsiflexion has more functional significance in stance than swing."

Look at Figure 2-5B-1. On it are depicted two patterns of excessive dorsiflexion. Explain both patterns:

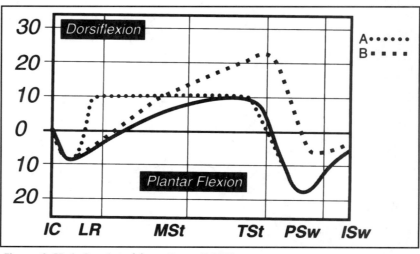

Figure 2-5B-1. Reprinted from Perry (1992).

Explanation of pattern A

Explanation of pattern B

2. Give three noncontractile problems that would result in excessive dorsiflexion. Explain your answers.

   a.

   b.

   c.

3. Give two contractile problems that would result in excessive dorsiflexion. Explain your answers.

   a.

   b.

4. Your patient is wearing an ankle-foot orthosis with the ankle joint fixed in neutral. What kind of gait deviations will be caused by this appliance?

   Describe the gait deviations as specifically as possible.

5. Describe one problem at the knee that will cause excessive dorsiflexion at the ankle.

Section C

Foot Deformities and Gait Deviations—Sagittal Plane

For each of the following foot deformities, describe the gait deviations that you would expect to see. Specify when in the gait cycle the deviations will occur.

   1. Pes cavus

   2. Equinus

   3. Talipes calcaneus

   4. Pes planus

Section D

Foot Deformities and Gait Deviations—Frontal Plane

For each of the following foot deformities, describe the gait deviations that you would expect to see. Specify when in the gait cycle the deviations will occur.

   1. Hindfoot varus

   2. Forefoot varus

   3. Forefoot valgus

Section E

Foot Deformities and Gait Deviations—Triplanar

For each of the following foot conditions, describe the gait deviations that you would expect to see. Specify when in the gait cycle the deviations will occur.

1. Equinovarus

2. Forefoot supinatus

3. Hindfoot varus with a forefoot supinatus

4. Hyperpronation

5. HAV

Section F

Gait Deviations

Define the following gait deviations (Figure 2-5F-1). Tell when you would observe them in the gait cycle, list the most likely causes, and describe the significance of these problems.

Problem	Definition	Phase of Gait Cycle	Cause(s)	Significance
Gait Deviation Table				
1. Foot slap				
2. Forefoot or foot-flat contact				
3. Excessive dorsiflexion				
4. Delayed heel contact				
5. Premature heel rise				
6. Prolonged heel contact (or delayed heel rise)				
7. Hyperpronation				
8. Excessive hindfoot supination				
9. Medial heel whip				
10. Lateral heel whip				
11. Foot or toe drag				
12. No heel off				
13. Vaulting over contralateral limb				
14. Toes up (dorsiflexed)				
15. Claw toes				

Figure 2-5F-1.

Section G

Sensory Factors

1. List as many causes as you can that would result in absent or decreased sensation in the foot.

2. What clinical signs and symptoms would lead you to suspect that your patient may have absent or decreased sensation? List as many as you can.

3. Hypersensitivity in the foot can also lead to gait deviations. Give two clinical examples.

4. Pain can produce the following gait deviations. Explain each one and give a clinical example.
   a. Shortened step length on involved side.

   b. Decreased ankle ROM with the joint held in 15° of plantarflexion.

   c. Decreased muscle strength.

Section H

Motor Control Deficits

Perry (1992) described five functional deficits that occur in patients with central neurological lesions (brain or spinal cord). Explain how each of these deficits can affect a patient's gait and describe how we can recognize each deficit while doing an observational gait analysis.

1. Spasticity and clonus.

2. Lack of selective muscle control.

3. Primitive locomotor patterns (e.g., mass flexion and mass extension).

4. Inappropriate phasing of muscle activation.

5. Sensory deficits and inadequate sensory feedback.

Part 6. Observational Gait Analysis—The Foot and Ankle

Designate one member of your lab group to be the walker and the rest of the group will be the analyzers.

Section A

History

Does the walker have a significant history of foot and ankle problems? *Yes.* ① *11/960: stress fracture in right big toe.*
pain under big toe; prescribed orthodics by podiatrist.
② *Knee problem - 1981 high school; orthodics kept her from pronating too much; knee still hurts when she*
If so, what is the problem? *runs.* ③ *rt. leg longer than left.*

List of relevant factors.

Section B

Physical Evaluation—Non-weight Bearing

Have the walker remove his or her shoes and socks and sit so both feet can be easily evaluated.
Unless otherwise noted, the following evaluation procedures are done bilaterally.

1. Observation *of Una.*

   Is the skin in good condition? *yes.*

   Note areas of redness, discoloration of skin and nail beds, break-down, edema, etc. *None*

   Do you see any obvious deformities? Note foot alignment. *Normal is inverted, plantarflexed, & adducted.*

   pt. prone

   Hindfoot alignment: varus, neutral, valgus. *Look @ calcaneus; medial aspect lower (valgus)*

1/98

ask Nancy ⟵ Forefoot alignment: plantarflexus, dorsiflexus, adductus, abductus, varus,
wood

   valgus, supinatus, pronatus.

   Describe any significant findings.

   Note location and condition of any (calluses,) corns, bunions, or other skin lesions. *left. foot* *right foot*
   3,4,5 digits *4, 5 digits*

   Are there any toe amputations? *no*

   Other: Note any other observations that appear significant. *No*

2. Active ROM—Ask the walker to actively dorsiflex and plantarflex each ankle, supinate and pronate each
   foot, and wiggle all of the toes. Note any limitations of motion, pain, or motor control abnormalities.
   Active ROM provides therapists with information about their patient's comprehension and their willing-
   ness to cooperate with the evaluation.

3. Passive ROM—This movement provides therapists with information about the noncontractile structures such
   as ligaments, fascia, joint capsules, etc. For each movement, note the range of motion and the end-feel.

   Talocrural: dorsiflexion and plantarflexion.

   Subtalar: supination and pronation.

   Transverse tarsal: dorsiflexion, plantarflexion, adduction, abduction, inversion, eversion.

   Mobilize all rays: superior and inferior glides.

   Metatarsalphalangeal (MTP) joints: dorsiflexion and plantarflexion.

   All proximal interphalangeal and distal interphalangeal joints: dorsiflexion and plantarflexion.

(I also include a test of the subtalar conversion mechanism. I sit in front of my patient and grasp the calcaneus with one hand and position my other hand under the metatarsal heads. I maximally pronate the calcaneus and lift up on the metatarsal heads. A certain amount of joint play should be possible. I maximally supinate the heel and lift up on the metatarsal heads. The joints of the midfoot should be in their close-packed positions and no motion should be possible.)

4. Resistive tests by muscle—see an appropriate muscles testing guide. This will provide information about the contractile structures.

5. Special tests—consult with an appropriate orthopedic text for the following tests:

      Bone spur/plantar fasciitis   Pitting/blanching

      Babinski's sign   Skin temperature

      Homans' sign   Sensation

Section C

Static Posture

Consult with appropriate sources for a posture evaluation.

      Sagittal—ear lobe; acromion; and trochanter, knee, and ankle line.

      Frontal—bilateral symmetry.

      Compare the arches of the feet in a weight-bearing situation with the nonweight-bearing condition.

      Comment on the hindfoot, midfoot, and forefoot alignment.

Section D

Foot and Ankle Gait Analysis

Walker should be barefoot with both feet visible.

1. Sagittal plane analysis—Observe the walker in the sagittal plane. Concentrate observations on one foot at a time.

    a. Initial contact—Does the foot demonstrate an appropriate heel strike? If not, describe the foot contact.

       Possible gait deviations:

          forefoot contact

          foot-flat contact

          step length problems

          toes exhibiting abnormal
            position or motion

    b. Loading response—Does the foot achieve an appropriate foot-flat position?

       Possible gait deviations:

foot slap	hindfoot and midfoot hyperpronation
wobble	toes up
initiation of primitive	toes clawed
extension pattern	vault to clear contralateral limb
excessive plantarflexion	(will be seen throughout stance phase)
excessive dorsiflexion	heel off
inadequate toe extension	hindfoot supination

c. Single limb support—Does the shin advance over the fixed foot in a controlled manner? Does the heel rise at the appropriate time in terminal stance?
Possible gait deviations:

excessive plantarflexion	no heel off
excessive dorsiflexion	toes clawed
hyperpronation	toes up
excessive supination	inadequate toe extension
early heel rise	

d. Preswing—Does the foot plantarflex and clear the floor?
Possible gait deviations:

excessive plantarflexion	no heel off
excessive dorsiflexion	toes clawed
hyperpronation	toes up
excessive supination	inadequate toe extension
medial heel whip — me	lateral heel whip

e. Swing phase—Does the foot clear the ground?
Possible gait deviations:

excessive plantarflexion	foot drag
excessive dorsiflexion	toe drag
hyperpronation	toes clawed
excessive supination	toes up

2. Frontal plane analysis—Observe the walker in the frontal plane. Concentrate observations on one foot at a time. Draw a line bisecting the walker's heels to help visualize hindfoot alignment.

a. Initial contact and loading response
Possible gait deviations:

wobble	vaulting to clear contralateral limb
hyperpronation	(will be seen throughout stance phase)
excessive supination	decreased or increased width of
	base of support (BOS)

b. Single limb support

Possible gait deviations:

hyperpronation   excessive toe-out

excessive supination   excessive toe-in

vaulting to clear contralateral limb

c. Preswing

Possible gait deviations:

medial heel whip

lateral heel whip

d. Swing phase

Possible gait deviations:

foot or toe drag   hyperpronation

excessive plantarflexion   excessive supination

excessive dorsiflexion

Part 7. Thought Questions

Section A

hallus abductus valgus

1. What is the relationship between HAV and hindfoot varus and hyperpronation?

2. If your patient has a leg length discrepancy, what gait deviations would you expect to see on the involved side and when in the gait cycle would they occur?

3. What is the windlass phenomenon?
   Explain the relationship between a claw toe deformity and a pes cavus.

4. For each of the foot/floor contact patterns in Figures 2-7A-1, 2-7A-2, and 2-7A-3, on the next page, identify at least one clinical problem that would cause this gait deviation.
   Briefly explain your answers.

Nancy Wood examined Mark's feet to show us some stuff. Great toe extension - 65° need for push off.
medial corns   weight-bearing = relaxed stance: look for forefoot ab/ad
callous on side of 5th digit   Knees - look @ tibia, arches, any bunyons
passively dorsiflex w/ knee straight   mark has valgus (hindfoot)
   ① invert calcaneous → should lock up mid-tarsal joint / then try to move foot into
inversion / eversion, ab/ad.
38
   ③ pronate calcaneous : open-pack position - unlock joint - should move better.
   ④ foot supinates: closed-pack position - lock up - less motion in sup than pron.
Look @ rays: 2,3,4 move together. 5 has its own. Can't up about

a. Clinical cause

b. Explanation

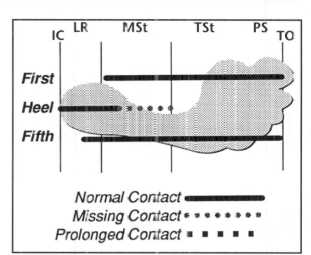

Figure 2-7A-1. Reprinted from Perry (1992).

a. Clinical cause

b. Explanation

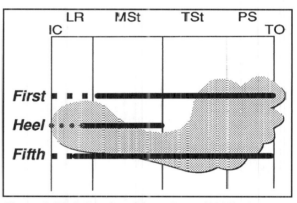

Figure 2-7A-2. Reprinted from Perry (1992). See Figure 2-7A-3 for key.

a. Clinical cause

b. Explanation

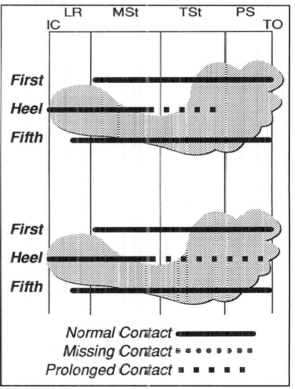

Figure 2-7A-3. Reprinted from Perry (1992).

Part 8. Video Gait Analysis—The Foot and Ankle

Add a new section to your gait form for recording your analysis of foot and ankle kinematics and kinetics. The foot and ankle section should follow the section on gait characteristics in the "O" part of your form. Now that you have had some experience with observing gait, you may want to revise your section on gait characteristics to better guide your observations. Use your revised form to analyze the gait of a new walker. Your assignment is to analyze the walker's gait characteristics and foot and ankle function in both the sagittal and frontal planes.

In the companion videotape, *People walking: Pathological patterns and normal changes over the life span*, Walker 2 in the first section of the tape can be used for this assignment. Her history is as follows.

Walker 2. Age 50 — video shown 2/4/98

Hallus Abductus Valgus

Walker 2 has a history of a fractured left fibula 10 years prior and bilateral plantar fasciitis with a left calcaneal heel spur 2 months before the filming. She has bilateral HAV and reports that she is starting to develop patellofemoral pain in the right knee.

on calcaneus on plantar aspect.

feet

normal step length
— 2.1 ft.

step - heel to heel

normal stride length
— 4.2 ft.
heel strike to heel strike

speed
— normal cadence 120 steps/minute

head position — looking down
trunk shifted back

no heel strike
low arch

rigid lever arm — you need this b/c as you walk forward
supinate - Tst.
pronation - unlocked so shock absorbing
Tibia rolls over talus & locks forefoot

if Don't lock up — in pronation too long so plantar fascia (helps to support arch)
this stretches the bundl of tissue that runs along bottom.
plantar fascia
avoid putting stress on plantar fascia so she doesn't hyperextend her toe that much.

heel spur — fascia gets irritated / plantar fascia pulling
blood, inflammation.
Wolf law — lay down bone in response to stress.

Knees

she lands on a pretty straight knee.
rt. knee — valgus thrust (knee pops in)
— when she is loading.

rt. hip abducts
rt. knee adducts
→ b/c of valgus thrust

The foot relates to the knee

little arm swing so little trunk rotation — these things help w/ momentum.
if she did longer stride maybe she would get more trunk movement.
rt. shoulder drops.

?? loose-packed
closed-packed.

Chapter Three

Normal and Pathological Knee Function

Objectives

1. To describe and analyze normal function of the knee during the gait cycle.
2. To recall the gait determinants previously presented.
3. To demonstrate an increased understanding of gait analysis.
4. To discuss gait deviations of the knee and their underlying causes.

Part 1. Terminology

6 degrees of freedom in knee

Section A

Motions of the Knee

Define the following terms:

1. Flexion — thigh & calf come closer together by bending the knee.

2. Extension — thigh & calf move farther apart.
   tr·

3. Internal (medial) rotation — knee rotates toward the midline.
   transverse plane motion

4. External (lateral) rotation — " " away from midline.
   transverse plane motion

5. Adduction — frontal plane motion; segment toward midline

6. Abduction — " " " " away from midline.

Section B
Deformities of the Knee

Define the following terms:

1. Genu varus – *knee in abduction bowlegs*

2. Genu valgum – *knee in adduction knock knees*

3. Genu recurvatum – *hyper extended knees*

4. Patella alta – *a high sitting patella*

5. Osgood-Schlatter disease – *enlarged tibial tubercle.*

Part 2. Normal Functional Anatomy

Section A
Osteology

1. Label the parts of the knee joint indicated in Figure 3-2A-1.

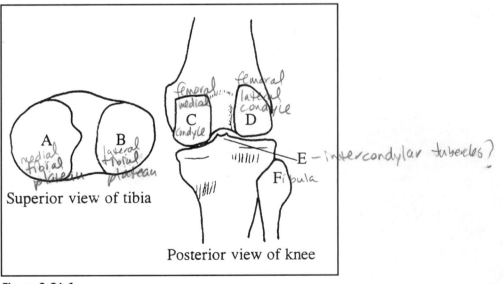

Figure 3-2A-1.

2. What is the close-packed position of the knee? *extension*

3. The medial tibial plateau is larger than the lateral tibial plateau. How does this affect knee function? *allows int/ext. rotation, & gliding of femoral condyles on tibial plateau*

4. Describe the *screw home* mechanism.
Femur rotates medially on tibia until full ext is achieved

valgus - knock kneed.

5. What role does the patella play in knee function? ↑ *lever arm ; mechanically sufficient.*

6. In adults, the long axis of the femur creates a physiological valgus at the knee. What are the implications of this alignment for gait? *....*

Section B

Arthrology

1. What is the capsular pattern of the knee? *more limitation in flex. than ext.*

2. What are the functions of the following structures?

a. The menisci - *deepen the articular surfaces of the tibia where they articulate w/ femoral condyles ; shock absorbers ; reduce friction.*

b. The anterior cruciate ligament - *do not allow ant. displacement of tibia*

c. The posterior cruciate ligament - *do not allow post* " " "

d. The medial collateral ligament - *does not allow excessive lat. rot. of tibia most effective in knee flex. stops joint from gapping on this side.*

e. The lateral collateral ligament - *...*

f. The coronary ligament - *bind the menisci to the tibial plateau.*

Section C

Osteokinematics and Arthrokinematics

1. The knee functions like a modified hinge joint. The modification results from the movement of the tibiofemoral joint axis during range of motion (ROM). Describe the movement of this axis as the knee goes from full extension to full flexion. *Axis of rotation is not where pin is (that would be a hinge joint)* *Axis of rotation moves b/c knee does not function w/ 1° of freedom. It changes as the knee moves.*

2. On Figure 3-2C-1, use an arrow to demonstrate which way the femur is moving on the tibia. To maintain osseous congruency as the knee moves, the femur slides on the tibial plateau in addition to rolling.

a. Which way does the femur slide and roll when the knee is flexing? *rolls post glides ant.*

b. Which way does the femur slide and roll when the knee is extending? *rolls ant. glides post.*

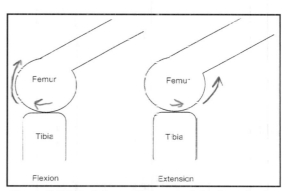

Figure 3-2C-1. Schematic views of the knee in the sagittal plane.

43

3. The femur rotates on the tibia around a longitudinal axis as the knee moves.

    a. Which way does the femur rotate when the knee is flexing? *laterally*

    b. Which way does the femur rotate when the knee is extending? *medially*

4. The tibiofemoral joint axis is not parallel to the ground but is slightly lower on the medial side. This obliquity causes a slight adduction and abduction of the lower leg as the knee goes through its ROM.

    a. With the femur fixed and the knee flexing, the lower leg demonstrates what frontal plane motion? *adducts*

    b. With the femur fixed and the knee extending, the lower leg demonstrates what frontal plane motion? *abducts*

Part 3. Normal Knee Function—Sagittal Plane

Section A

Kinematics

Look → p.129 – Subdivisions of gait cycle.

In Figure 3-3A-1 showing knee ROM, draw in the curve that describes the movement of the knee joint during the gait cycle.

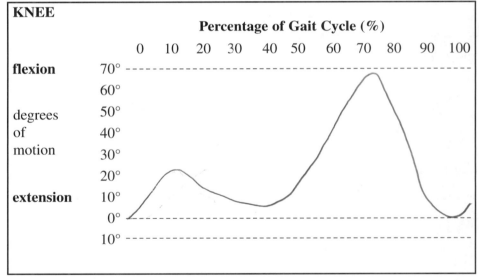

Figure 3-3A-1.

Section B

Kinetics

On Figures 3-3B-1, 3-3B-2, 3-3B-3, and 3-3B-4, label each electromyogram (EMG) tracing with the name of the appropriate muscles. Gray areas indicate variations in muscle activation between subjects.

PSw- weight off foot
ISw- foot moving.

Muscle Name

Don't compare one to the other in magnitude.

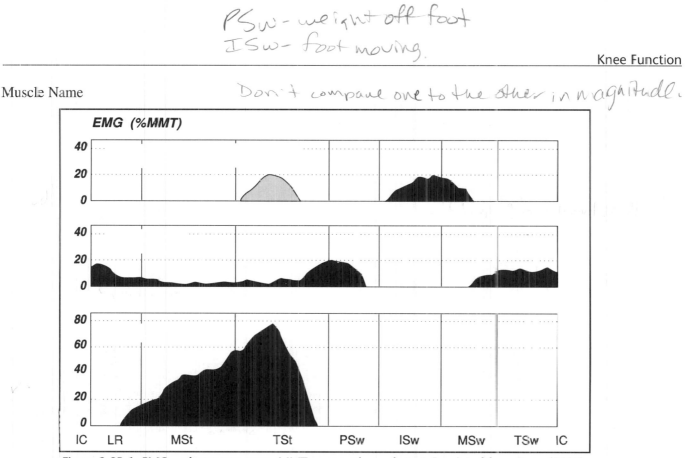

Figure 3-3B-1. EMG = electromyogram; MMT = manual muscle test. Reprinted from Perry (1992).

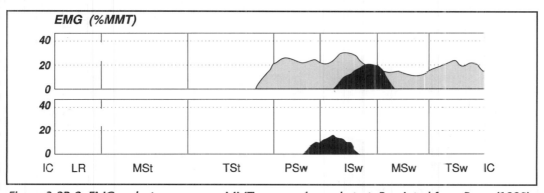

Figure 3-3B-2. EMG = electromyogram; MMT = manual muscle test. Reprinted from Perry (1992).

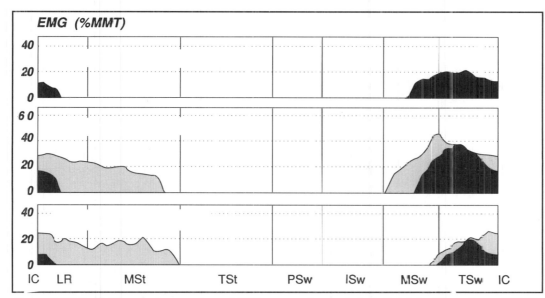

Figure 3-3B-3. EMG = electromyogram; MMT = manual muscle test. Reprinted from Perry (1992).

Muscle Name

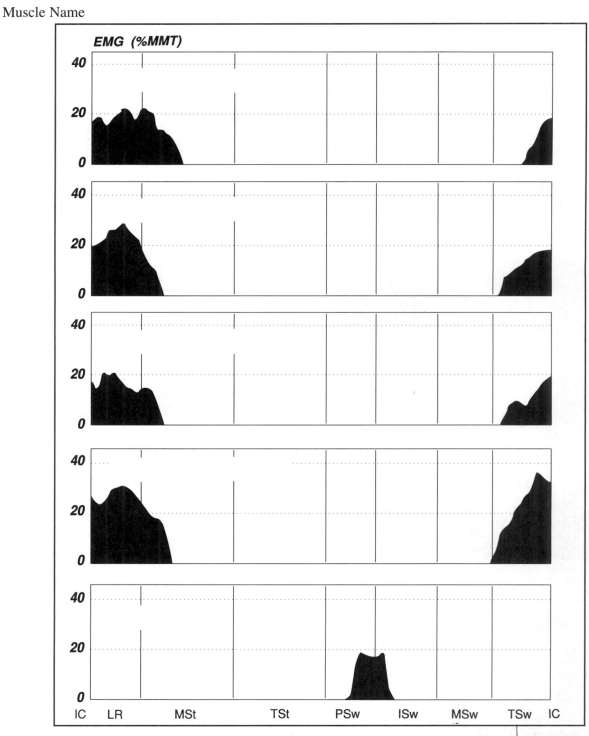

Figure 3-3B-4. EMG = electromyogram; MMT = manual muscle test. Reprinted from Perry (1992).

Concentric

During which of the subdivision(s) of gait do the following occur (Figure 3-3B-5).

Gait Subdivision Table	
1. Maximal knee flexion (ROM)	ISw
2. Maximal knee extension (ROM)	TSw
3. Extensor muscle activity manual muscle test (MMT)	heel strike, foot flat,
4. Flexor muscle activity (MMT)	

Figure 3-3B-5.

5. On Figure 3-3B-6, draw in the muscle groups that are active during each subdivision of stance phase. Explain the relationship between the position of the knee (ROM) and the activation of specific muscle groups (EMG). Include in your answer consideration of the vector forces illustrated by the sequence of pictures.

Explanation

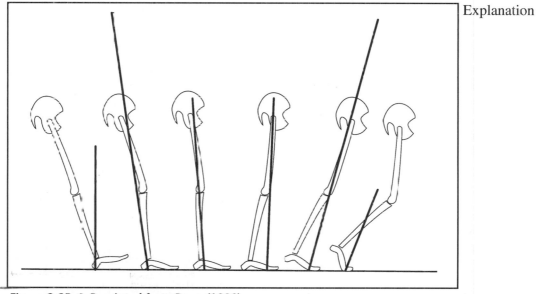

Figure 3-3B-6. Reprinted from Perry (1992).

Part 4. Normal Knee Function—Transverse Plane

The lower limb internally and externally rotates during the gait cycle. Starting with initial contact (IC), describe the transverse plane kinematics of the knee. Include in your explanation when the limb is maximally internally rotated, when it is maximally externally rotated, and what the ROM is at the knee in the transverse plane.

What function do you think the biceps femoris plays at the knee in the transverse plane?

Part 5. Normal Knee Function—Frontal Plane

Research shows that a slight amount (8°) of abduction and adduction occurs at the knee joint during gait (Kettlecamp, Johnson, Smidt, Chao, & Walker, 1970).

1. During which of the subdivisions of gait does knee abduction occur?

2. During which of the subdivisions of gait does knee adduction occur?

3. What role does the iliotibial band play at the knee in the frontal plane?

Part 6. Knee Pathomechanics

Section A

Kinetics

In Figure 3-6A-1 showing knee ROM, copy the graph you drew in Part 3. Now put a star on the graph for the following subdivisions of gait: loading response (LR), midstance (MSt), pre-swing (PSw), initial swing (ISw) and terminal swing (TSw). These are the parts of the gait cycle where abnormal knee function is most significant.

KNEE		Percentage of Gait Cycle (%)										
		0	10	20	30	40	50	60	70	80	90	100
flexion	70°	---										
	60°											
degrees	50°											
of	40°											
motion	30°											
	20°											
extension	10°											
	0°	---										
	10°	---										

Figure 3-6A-1.

Section B

Specific Gait Deviations

A. *Inadequate flexion* is defined as a failure of the knee to accomplish the normal amount of flexion resulting in limited or absent motion. Pathologically, we can see inadequate knee flexion during LR, ISw, and PSw. In your group, demonstrate the gait of someone who has inadequate knee flexion. First demonstrate the gait unilaterally, then bilaterally.

1. Describe the difference between the unilateral and bilateral gait deviations.

2. What role does normal knee flexion play during these periods of the gait cycle that a patient with inadequate knee flexion lacks?

3. List two noncontractile reasons for inadequate knee flexion.
   inability to "
   a. bony problem
   b.

4. List two contractile reasons for inadequate knee flexion.
   a. joint contracture
   b.

B. *Excessive extension* is defined as motion of the knee beyond neutral (> 0° extension). This problem can be seen clinically as either an *extensor thrust* or a *hyperextension*. *Extensor thrust* is defined as an excessive extensor force when the knee lacks hyperextension range. Extensor thrust can be seen during MSt. Demonstrate this gait problem. First demonstrate the gait unilaterally, then bilaterally.
   weak quads, so you would hyperextend.

1. Describe the difference between these two gait deviations.

2. Give two reasons for extensor thrust.
   a.
   b.

C. *Hyperextension* occurs when the knee joint angulates posteriorly (recurvatum). This can be seen clinically during any weight-bearing subdivision of gait. Hyperextension can be slow and passive or fast and active. Demonstrate this type of gait problem. First demonstrate the gait unilaterally, then bilaterally.

1. Describe the difference between these two gait deviations.

2. Give an active and a passive reason for the knee to hyperextend.

    a. Passive reason

    b. Active reason

D. *Excessive flexion* means that the knee has more than the normal range of flexion for that period in the gait cycle. We see this problem during LR and MSw. Demonstrate excessive knee flexion. First demonstrate the gait unilaterally, then bilaterally. Describe the difference between these two gait deviations. List the four major reasons for *excessive knee flexion*.

1. Describe the differences between the two gaits.

2. List four causes of excessive knee flexion.

    a.

    b.

    c.

    d.

E. *Inadequate extension* can be defined as persistent flexion at a time when knee extension is normally occurring. This problem is seen during MSt and TSw. Demonstrate this gait deviation. First demonstrate the gait unilaterally, then bilaterally.

1. Describe the difference between these two gait deviations.

2. List four reasons for inadequate knee extension.

    a.

    b.

    c.

    d.

B. Frontal plane knee problems include excessive varus or valgus. Both can result from static or dynamic influences. Patients often display a mixture of these two mechanisms. Complete Figure 3-6B-1 to better understand frontal plane problems of the knee. List as many factors as you can. As you list each factor, consider how you would test for this problem in the clinic.

Frontal Plane Knee Problems Table		
Static Factors	**Dynamic Factors**	**Clinical Tests**
1. Excessive varus		
2. Excessive valgus		

Figure 3-6B-1.

Part 7. Clinical Gait Deviations

Section A

Demonstrate the gait deviations in Figure 3-7A-1, and then complete the table indicating when during the gait cycle you would expect to see the problem, its most likely cause, and its significance.

Clinical Gait Deviations Table			
Gait Deviation	**When Seen in Gait Cycle**	**Cause**	**Significance**
1. Inadequate flexion			
2. Excessive flexion			
3. Inadequate extension			
4. Hyperextension			
5. Extensor thrust			
6. Wobble or buckling			
7. Excessive flexion as a contralateral compensation			

Figure 3-7A-1.

Part 8. Observational Gait Analysis—The Knee

Choose one member of your lab group to be the walker. The walker should be wearing appropriate clothing so that the people doing the gait analysis can see both knees, thighs, shins, ankles, and feet. Before doing a gait analysis, it is appropriate to take a case history, do an orthopedic knee evaluation, and perform a static postural analysis.

Section A

Sagittal Plane

Observe one knee at a time in the sagittal plane.

1. Weight acceptance (IC and LR)—Was the knee close to full extension (-5°) at initial contact? Did the knee flex during LR?

   Possible gait deviations:

   excessive or limited knee flexion
   hyperextension
   extensor thrust
   wobbling
   buckling

2. Single limb support—Is the knee extending until heel rise when flexion occurs?

   Possible gait deviations:

   inadequate extension
   hyperextension
   extensor thrust
   wobbling
   buckling

3. Preswing—Is the knee flexing to clear the foot?

   Possible gait deviations:

   inadequate or excessive flexion
   hyperextension
   extensor thrust

4. Swing phase—In early swing, is the knee flexing to clear foot? In late swing, is the knee extending to prepare for IC?

   Possible gait deviations:

   early swing: inadequate or excessive knee flexion
   late swing: inadequate extension, hyperextension, extensor thrust
   swing phase: excessive knee flexion throughout to compensate for short contralateral limb

Section B
Frontal Plane

Observe one knee at a time in the frontal plane.

1. Stance phase

>   Possible gait deviations

>>   excessive abduction or adduction
>>   excessive internal or external rotation

2. Swing phase

>   Possible gait deviations

>>   excessive abduction or adduction

Part 9. Thought Questions

1. During gait the soleus muscle functions to extend the knee. Explain how this works.

2. Women athletes tend to have a much greater incidence of knee injuries in weight-bearing sports than men. Discuss the effects of an increased Q angle on knee injury.

3. Your patient has bilateral 45° knee flexion contractures. Describe the compensations you would expect to see at this patient's hips, pelvic girdle, and dorsal spine when viewing the patient standing in the sagittal plane.

    Diagram this patient's posture to illustrate your answer.

4. Your patient has severe rheumatoid arthritis of both knees resulting in bilateral genu valgum. Both knees are hot, swollen, and painful.

    a. What is the resting position for knees in this condition?

    b. Describe the kinds of gait deviations you would expect this patient to exhibit at the knee. Explain your answer.

c. Bilateral genu valgum will cause what kind of compensations at the foot and ankle?

d. Describe the foot and ankle gait deviations you expect this patient to demonstrate.

e. Bilateral genu valgum will cause what kind of compensations at the hip, pelvis, and trunk? Describe these gait deviations.

5. Genu recurvatum will cause what kind of compensations at the foot and ankle?

   Genu recurvatum will cause what kind of alignment compensations at the hip, pelvis, and trunk?

6. Describe the alignment compensations that can be expected at the foot and ankle, hip, pelvis, and trunk in a patient with bilateral genu varum.

7. Your patient has a loose body in one knee. What kind of gait deviations will this person demonstrate? Be as specific as you can. Explain your answer.

8. You have a patient with a torn medial meniscus. What kind of gait deviations will this person demonstrate? Be as specific as you can. Explain your answer.

Part 10. Video Gait Analysis—The Knee

Add a new section to your gait form for recording your analysis of knee kinematics and kinetics. The knee section should follow the section on the foot and ankle in the "O" part of your form. You may want to revise your previous sections to better guide your observations. Use your revised form to analyze the gait of a new walker. Your assignment is to analyze the walker's gait characteristics, foot and ankle function, and knee function in both the sagittal and frontal planes.

In the companion videotape, *People walking: Pathological patterns and normal changes over the life span*, Patient 3 in the first section of the tape can be used for this assignment. Her history is as follows.

Walker 3. Age 31

Walker 3 has a history of rheumatoid arthritis in her neck, hips, knees, and feet. She had a C_{1-2} fusion and fluid removed from her knees.

Chapter Four

Normal and Pathological Hip Function

Objectives

1. To describe and analyze normal hip joint function during the gait cycle.
2. To recall the gait determinants previously presented.
3. To demonstrate an increased understanding of gait analysis.
4. To discuss gait deviations of the hip and their underlying causes.

Part 1. Terminology

Section A
Motions of the Hip

Define the following terms:

1. Flexion

2. Extension

3. Internal (medial) rotation

4. External (lateral) rotation

5. Adduction

6. Abduction

Section B

Deformities of the Hip

Define the following terms and label the bones according to their deformities:

1. Coxa vara (Figure 4-1B-1)

2. Coxa valga (Figure 4-1B-1)

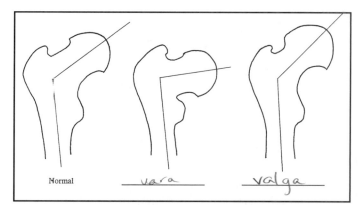

Figure 4-1B-1. The proximal aspect of the femur in the frontal plane.

3. Anteversion (Figure 4-1B-2)

look in Magee
normal femoral ↗ 8-15°
anteversion is ↑

4. Retroversion (Figure 4-1B-2)

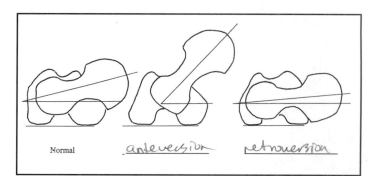

Figure 4-1B-2. A transverse plane representation of the femur showing the head, greater trochanter, and femoral condyles.

Define the following terms:

5. Legg-Calvé-Perthes disease

6. Slipped capital epiphysis

7. Congenital hip dislocation

Ober Test- iliotibial band test. Abduct leg & a little extension tight hip flexors (iliopsoas)

Part 2. Normal Functional Anatomy

Section A
Osteology

1. Label the structures indicated on the acetabulum and proximal femur in Figures 4-2A-1 and 4-2A-2.

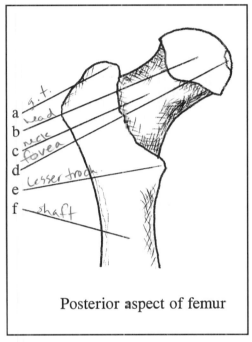

a _g.t._
b _head_
c _neck_
d _fovea_
e _lesser troch_
f _shaft_

Posterior aspect of femur

Figure 4-2A-1.

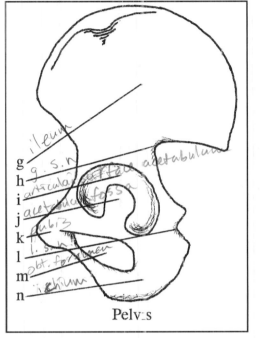

g _ileum_
h _g.s.n_
i _articular_
j _acetab fossa_
k _pubis_
l _s.n_
m _obt. foramen_
n _ischium_

Pelvis

Figure 4-2A-2.

2. Define the following terms:
   a. Angle of inclination

   b. Angle of torsion

   c. Trabeculae

   d. Zone of weakness

Section B
Arthrology

1. What is the close-packed position of the hip joint?

2. What is the position of maximal articular congruency?

3. What is the function of the ligamentum teres?

4. What kind of joint is the hip joint and how many degrees of freedom does it have?

5. What ligaments support the hip joint anteriorly?

6. What ligaments support the hip joint posteriorly?

Part 3. Hip Movements and the Closed Kinematic Chain

Section A
Pelvic Girdle and Lumbar Spine Responses

The hip joint is closely linked to the pelvic girdle and the lumbar spine. In a closed chain configuration, movement of the hip joint results in specific movements of the pelvic girdle and the lumbar spine. Discover these movements for yourself by performing the hip movements below while standing on the designated limb. Record your observations of the pelvic girdle and the lumbar spine responses in Figure 4-3A-1.

Response Table		
Hip Movements	**Pelvic Girdle Responses**	**Lumbar Spine Responses**
1. Flexion		
2. Extension		
3. Abduction		
4. Adduction		
5. Internal (medial) Rotation		
6. External (lateral) Rotation		

Figure 4-3A-1.

Section B

Knee, Ankle, and Foot Responses

Perform the same hip movements again while standing on the designated limb and record the responses occurring at the knee, ankle, and foot in Figure 4-3B-1.

Hip Movements	Response Table Knee Responses	Ankle and Foot Responses
1. Flexion		
2. Extension		
3. Abduction		
4. Adduction		
5. Internal (medial) Rotation		
6. External (lateral) Rotation		

Figure 4-3B-1.

Part 4. Normal Hip Function—Sagittal Plane

Section A

Kinematics

On Figure 4-4A-1 showing hip range of motion (ROM), draw in the curve that describes the movement of the hip joint during the gait cycle.

HIP		Percentage of Gait Cycle (%)
		0 10 20 30 40 50 60 70 80 90 100
flexion	60°	
degrees	40°	
of	20°	
motion	0°	
extension	20°	
	40°	

Figure 4-4A-1.

Section B

Kinetics

On Figures 4-4B-1, 4-4B-2, 4-4B-3, and 4-4B-4, label each electromyogram (EMG) tracing with the name of the appropriate muscles. Gray areas indicate variations in muscle activation between subjects.

Muscle Names

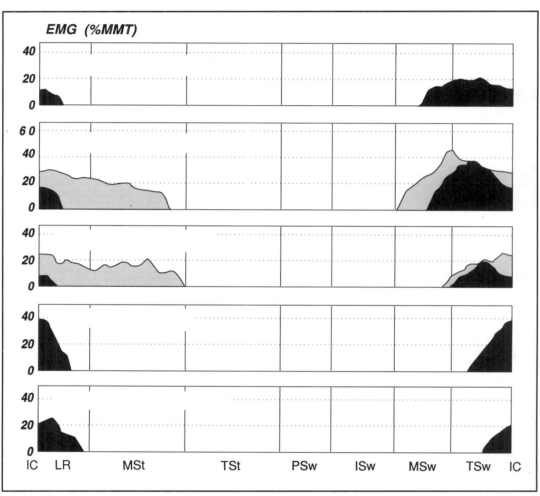

Figure 4-4B-1. EMG = electromyogram; MMT = manual muscle test. Reprinted from Perry (1992).

Muscle Names

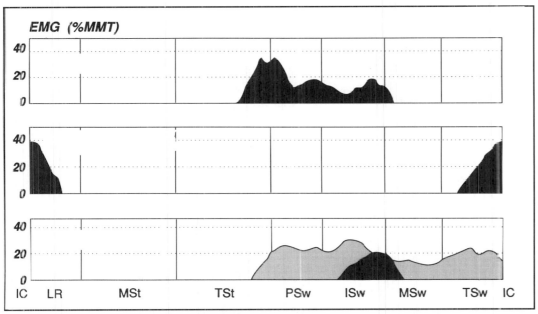

Figure 4-4B-2. EMG = electromyogram; MMT = manual muscle test. Reprinted from Perry (1992).

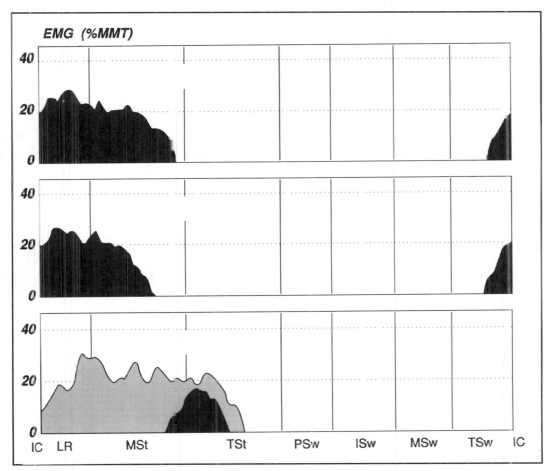

Figure 4-4B-3. EMG = electromyogram; MMT = manual muscle test. Reprinted from Perry (1992).

Muscle Names

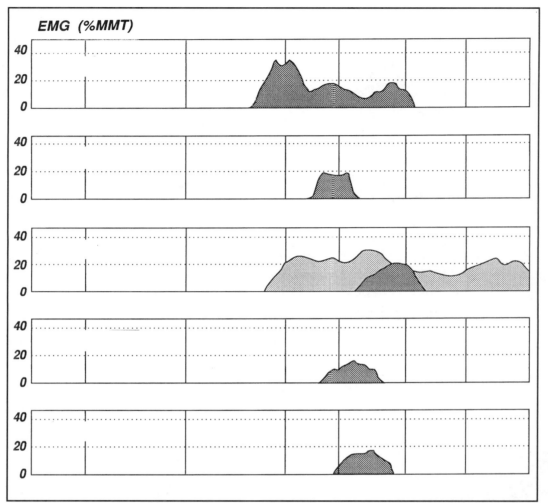

Figure 4-4B-4. EMG = electromyogram; MMT = manual muscle test. Reprinted from Perry (1992).

During which of the subdivision(s) of gait (Figure 4-4B-5) do the following occur?

See picture on p. 4.

Gait Subdivision Table
1. Maximal hip flexion (ROM)
2. Maximal hip extension (ROM)
3. Extensor muscle activity (MMT)
4. Flexor muscle activity (MMT)

Figure 4-4B-5.

5. Explain the relationship between the position of the hip (ROM) and the activation of specific muscle groups (EMG).

Part 5. Normal Hip Function—Frontal Plane

Section A

Research [Murray, Drought, & Kory (1964), Murray, Kory, & Sepic (1970)] shows that a small amount of abduction and adduction occur at the hip joint during gait. To see this motion, place masking tape on a subject horizontally from one anterior superior iliac spine (ASIS) to the other. Place a second piece of masking tape vertically on one leg from the superior border of the patella to the ASIS on that same side. Now watch the subject walk in the frontal plane.

1. During which subdivision of gait does maximal hip abduction occur?

2. During which subdivision of gait does maximal hip adduction occur?

3. On Figure 4-5A-1 showing hip ROM, draw in the curve that describes the movement of the hip joint during the gait cycle in the frontal plane.

HIP												
	Percentage of Gait Cycle (%)											
		0	10	20	30	40	50	60	70	80	90	100
	20°											
adduction	10°											
degrees	0°											
of motion	10°											
abduction	20°											

Figure 4-5A-1.

Part 6. Normal Hip Function—Transverse Plane

The lower limb internally (medially) and externally (laterally) rotates during the gait cycle. Starting with initial contact, describe the transverse plane kinematics of the hip. Include in your explanation when the limb is maximally internally rotated, when it is maximally externally rotated, and what the ROM is at the hip in the transverse plane.

What factors cause this transverse plane motion?

Part 7. Hip Pathomechanics

In Figure 4-7A-1 showing hip ROM, copy the graph you drew in Part 1. Now put a star on the graph on the parts of the gait cycle where abnormal hip function is most significant.

HIP												
		Percentage of Gait Cycle (%)										
		0	10	20	30	40	50	60	70	80	90	100
flexion	60°	--										
	40°											
degrees	20°	--										
of												
motion	0°											
	20°											
extension	40°	--										

Figure 4-7A-1.

Section A

Inadequate extension can be defined as persistent flexion at a time when hip extension is normally occurring.

1. During which part(s) of the gait cycle is the hip in its extension range?

2. Demonstrate the gait deviation of inadequate hip extension, first unilaterally, then bilaterally.

3. List as many causes for inadequate hip extension as you can.

Section B

Excessive flexion means that the hip has more than the normal range of flexion for that period in the gait cycle.

1. Demonstrate excessive hip flexion. First demonstrate the gait unilaterally, then bilaterally. What is the difference between inadequate hip extension and excessive hip flexion?

2. List as many causes for excessive hip flexion as you can.

Section C

Inadequate flexion is defined as a failure of the hip to accomplish the normal amount of flexion resulting in limited or absent motion.

1 Look at your sagittal plane hip ROM chart. When is the hip flexing?

2. Look at the EMG tracings. When are the hip flexor muscles active?

3. In your group, demonstrate the gait of someone who has inadequate hip flexion. First demonstrate the gait unilaterally, then bilaterally. Describe the difference between these two gait deviations.

Section D

Other hip deviations in the sagittal plane. Clinically, we see many compensations at the hip for problems in other parts of the lower limb.

Describe the gait deviations you would expect to see at the hip for the following problems (include the appropriate subdivisions of the gait cycle):

1. Foot drop (dorsiflexors weak).

2. Quadriceps weak.

3. Fixed anterior pelvic tilt.

4. Fixed posterior pelvic tilt.

Section E

Hip problems in the frontal and transverse planes.

1. Recall your definition of coxa vara. What effect would this condition have on the knee, ankle, and foot if the head of the femur is fixed in the acetabulum? Explain your answer.

What effect would coxa vara have on the knee, ankle, and foot if the head of the femur is free to move in the acetabulum? Explain your answer.

65

2. Recall your definition of coxa valga. What effect would this condition have on the knee, ankle, and foot if the head of the femur is fixed in the acetabulum? Explain your answer.

   What effect would coxa vara have on the knee, ankle, and foot if the head of the femur is free to move in the acetabulum? Explain your answer.

3. Recall your definition of hip anteversion and explain the influence of this deformity on gait.

Section F

Clinical problems. Describe and demonstrate the gait deviation that you would expect to see with the following clinical problems:

1. Hip abductor (muscle) weakness

2. Hip adductor (muscle) contracture

3. Hip adductor (muscle) spasticity

4. Iliotibial band tightness

5. Knee flexion contracture

6. Severe pain (i.e., arthritis) in the joint. Include in your answer the position of least intra-articular pressure.

7. Explain why giving a patient a cane in the contralateral hand can relieve an antalgic limp.

8. Develop and describe a strategy for use during a gait analysis by which you can determine whether a clinical problem is arising at the hip joint, or whether you are seeing a compensation at the hip and the problem is somewhere else in the closed chain.

Part 8. Gait Deviations

Section A

Complete Figure 4-8A-1 for gait deviations that you may observe at the hip. For each problem, tell when it occurs in the gait cycle, its most likely cause, and its significance.

Hip Gait Deviations Table			
Problem	**When Seen in Gait Cycle**	**Cause**	**Significance**
1. Inadequate flexion			
2. Excessive flexion			
3. Inadequate extension			
4. Past thigh retraction			
5. Excessive internal rotation			
6. Excessive external rotation			
7. Excessive abduction			
8. Excessive adduction			

Figure 4-8A-1.

Part 9. Observational Gait Analysis—The Hip

Select one member of your lab group to be the walker. The walker should be wearing appropriate clothing so everyone analyzing the gait can see both thighs, both knees, both shins, both ankles, both feet, and the pelvic girdle. Gait analysis should be done with the walker barefoot. It is appropriate before doing a gait analysis to take a case history, perform an appropriate orthopedic examination of the hip, and assess the person's static posture.

Section A
Sagittal Plane Analysis

Analyze one hip at a time in the sagittal plane.

1. Weight acceptance (initial contact and loading response)—Is the hip held in approximately 25° to 30° of flexion to facilitate shock absorption?

   Possible gait deviations:

   excessive or inadequate flexion

2. Single limb support—Is the hip extending to approximately 20° of hyperextension just before heel rise?

   Possible gait deviation:

   inadequate extension

3. Preswing—As the heel rises, does the hip flex to help clear the foot and advance the limb?

   Possible gait deviations:

   inadequate flexion
   inadequate extension (if missing hyperextension in terminal stance)

4. Swing phase—Is the hip flexed to help clear the foot and advance the limb?

   Possible gait deviations:

   inadequate flexion
   excessive flexion
   past thigh retraction (terminal swing)

Section B
Frontal Plane

Analyze one hip at a time in the frontal plane.

   Possible gait deviations that can occur throughout the gait cycle:

      excessive or inadequate internal or external rotation
      excessive or inadequate
      abduction or adduction

Part 10. Thought Questions

Section A

You have a patient who sustained a complete L$_3$ lesion of the spinal cord.

1. What do we mean when we say an "L$_3$ lesion of the spinal cord"?

2. List all the muscles of the lower extremities that are still functioning in this patient.

3. This patient is at high risk for developing joint problems at the hips, knees, and ankles. For each of these joints, describe the problems that you expect to develop and explain your answer in Figure 4-10A-1.

Joint Problems Table		
Joint	Problem	Explanation
Hip		
Knee		
Ankle		

Figure 4-10A-1.

4. This patient wants to walk again. Design and describe a gait training program for this patient.

What kind of gait pattern would this patient have?

Is independent ambulation a reasonable goal?
List the factors you would consider when planning a program for this patient.

Part 11. Video Gait Analysis—The Hip

Add a new section to your gait form for recording your analysis of hip kinematics and kinetics. The hip section should follow the section on the knee in the "O" part of your form. You may want to revise your previous sections to better guide your observations. Use your revised form to analyze the gait of a new walker. Your assignment is to analyze the walker's gait characteristics, foot and ankle function, knee function, and hip function in both the sagittal and frontal planes.

In the companion videotape, *People walking: Pathological patterns and normal changes over the life span*, Walker 4 in the first section of the tape can be used for this assignment. His history is as follows.

Walker 4. Age 44 — 2/11/98 w/ Cynthia

Walker 4 has had a long history of low back pain and gait problems. Within the last 10 years, his right hip was diagnosed as the source of his musculoskeletal dysfunction and he is a candidate for a total hip replacement.

my own observation:

no heel strike on either foot
rt. leg turned out.
limb — does not keep weight on rt. side
left arm swings more
toes out
patellas out

Discussion:
Step length — 1½ on rt.
    he swings further w/ rt. foot than left foot.
more time spent on left leg.
early heel rise
no hip extension on rt.
no heel strike on left.
big left arm swing
hip hiking rt. leg
hip abductors weak or he feels pain. (antalgic gait)
                                        ∟ pain relieving gait.
toe-out position for wider BOS.
adducting
landing @ mid-foot — a lot of pronation.
adduction + flexion — pt. w/ hip pain prefers this position b/c open packed & can fit more
                        stuff within the space.

hip hiked to avoid using ilio-psoas b/c i.p. muscle goes over hip joint &
    this can cause pain.

Chapter Five

Normal and Pathological Kinematics and Kinetics— Head, Arms, and Torso

Objectives

1. To describe the normal function of the pelvis and trunk during the gait cycle.
2. To describe pathological gaits resulting from problems in the pelvis and trunk.
3. To discuss the normal function of the head and arms during the gait cycle.
4. To explain how pathologies in the lower extremities and axial skeleton can influence the upper extremity function during gait.
5. To demonstrate an increased understanding of selected pathological gaits.

Part 1. Normal Head, Arms, and Trunk Function

Elftman (1954) used the acronym HAT to designate the passenger unit. These initials stand for head, arms, and torso. The torso includes both the trunk and the pelvic girdle.

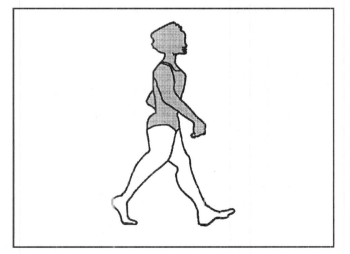

Figure 5-1A-1.

Section A
Displacement of the Center of Gravity

1. Recall the vertical displacement of the center of gravity (COG).
   a. When during the gait cycle is the COG the highest?
   b. When during the gait cycle is the COG the lowest?
   c. How much vertical displacement is normal?
   d. Describe four strategies that the body employs to minimize the vertical displacement of the COG.
      i.

      ii.

      iii.

      iv.

2. Recall the lateral displacement of the COG.
   a. When does the COG shift maximally to the right during the gait cycle?
   b. When does the COG shift maximally to the left during the gait cycle?
   c. How much lateral displacement is normal?
   d. Describe two strategies that the body employs to minimize the lateral displacement of the COG.
      i.

      ii.

Section B
Pelvic Girdle Movement

1. Recall the pelvic movements in three planes during gait:
   a. Sagittal
   b. Frontal
   c. Transverse

2. What is the normal range of motion (ROM) for pelvic motion in each plane during gait?
   a. Sagittal
   b. Frontal
   c. Transverse

d. Place masking tape from one anterior superior iliac spine (ASIS) to the other, from one posterior superior iliac spine (PSIS) to the other, and along both iliac crests of each member of your lab group. Watch the pelvic motions as each person walks. How do the pelvic motions of your lab partners compare with the norms? Explain your answer.

2. What happens to a person's gait cycle if pelvic motion is restricted? Write down your hypotheses.

Now try this experiment. You will need:
* *a 30-ft walkway*
* *a stop watch*
* *a lumbosacral orthosis*

Select one member of your lab group to be each of the following:
* *a walker*
* *a timer*
* *a step counter*
* *a sagittal plane pelvic motion analyzer*
* *a frontal plane pelvic motion analyzer*

On the designated walker, place masking tape from one ASIS to the other, from one PSIS to the other, and along both iliac crests. The walker will wait at the beginning of the walkway until the timer says, "Go." The walker will then walk down the walkway as the timer times the gait, the step counter counts the number of steps, and the two plane analyzers record what they see. Enter your findings in Figure 5-1B-1.

Pelvic Girdle Movement Table	
Time walker took to go 30 ft:	_____ sec
Velocity of walker:	_____ ft/sec
Number of steps walker took to go 30 ft:	_____ steps
Cadence:	_____ steps/sec
Analysis of pelvic motion in sagittal plane:	
Analysis of pelvic motion in frontal plane:	

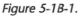
Figure 5-1B-1.

Now have the walker put on the lumbosacral orthosis and repeat the above procedure. Record your new findings in Figure 5-1B-2.

Pelvic Girdle Movement (With Orthosis) Table

Time walker took to go 30 ft: _____ sec

Velocity of walker: _____ ft/sec

Number of steps walker took to go 30 ft: _____ steps

Cadence: _____ steps/sec

Analysis of pelvic motion in sagittal plane:

Analysis of pelvic motion in frontal plane:

Figure 5-1B-2.

Compare the results of both trials. Did your results agree with your hypothesis?

Part 2. Shoulder Girdle and Upper Extremity Function

Section A

1. Observe shoulder girdle motion with respect to pelvic girdle motion in the frontal plane during gait. What is the relationship between these two? Explain why this relationship exists.

2. Upper extremity kinematics

On a member of your lab group, place masking tape on the midline of the trunk in the sagittal plane, on the midline of the humerus from the shoulder to the elbow and from the elbow to the wrist. Watch this person walk. On Figure 5-2A-1, draw in the curve that describes the movement of the shoulder and the elbow joints during the gait cycle.

ARM													
	Percentage of Gait Cycle (%)												
	0	10	20	30	40	50	60	70	80	90	100		
											Elbow		
flexion	50°												
	40°												
	30°												
degrees of motion	20°												
	10°												
	0°	- -												
	10°												
extension	20°											**Shoulder**		
	30°	- -												

Figure 5-2A-1.

3. Upper extremity kinetics

On Figure 5-2A-2, label each of the appropriate muscles. Choose from this list: middle deltoid, posterior deltoid, supraspinatus, teres major, upper trapezius.

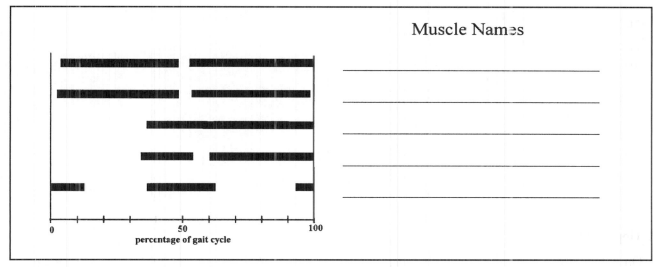

Figure 5-2A-2.

75

Part 3. Head, Arms, and Torso—Variations in Gait Parameters

Section A

Observing the Head, Arms, and Torso

Select a member of your lab group to be the walker. Have the walker demonstrate a normal gait pattern and then vary the gait parameters listed below. Describe the changes that you see in the HAT kinematics as you vary the following gait parameters:

- *increased step length on the right (R)*

- *decreased step time on the left (L)*

- *wide base of support (BOS)*

- *narrow BOS*

- *increased L toe-out*

- *decreased R toe-out*

- *increased cadence with no change in velocity*

- *increased cadence with decreased velocity*

- *decreased cadence with increased velocity*

- *increased velocity*

- *decreased velocity*

Record your observations in Figure 5-3A-1.

HAT Kinematics Table			
Gait Parameters	**Results Seen On**		
	Head	**Arm Swing**	**Torso**
Normal gait			
Increased step length on R			
Decreased step time on L			
Wide BOS			
Narrow BOS		·	
Increased L toe out			
Decreased R toe out			
Increased cadence with no change in velocity			
Increased cadence with decreased velocity			
Decreased cadence with increased velocity			
Increased velocity			
Decreased velocity			

Figure 5-3A-1.

Section B
Analysis

Based on your observations in the above section make some generalizations about the role in gait of the:

    1. Arm

2. Head

3. Trunk

4. Pelvic girdle

Part 4. Pathological Gaits

Section A

In your lab group, demonstrate and discuss the pathological gaits listed in Figure 5-4A-1. For each gait deviation, tell when in the gait cycle we would see the problem, its most likely cause, and its significance.

Pathological Gait Table

Gait Deviation	When Seen in Gait Cycle	Cause	Significance
1. Backward trunk lean			
2. Forward trunk lean			
3. Lateral trunk lean			
4. Trunk with backward rotation			
5. Trunk with forward rotation			
6. Increased lumbar lordosis			
7. Hip hiking			
8. Posterior pelvic tilt			
9. Anterior pelvic tilt			
10. Reduced or absent forward pelvic rotation			
11. Reduced or absent backward pelvic rotation			
12. Excessive backward pelvic rotation			
13. Ipsilateral pelvic drop			
14. Contralateral pelvic drop			

Figure 5-4A-1.

Part 5. Observational Gait Analysis—The Head, Arms, and Torso

Section A
Pelvic Motion in the Sagittal Plane

Select a member of your lab group to be a walker.

Analyze the walker's pelvic motion in the sagittal plane. Mark the walker's iliac crests with masking tape to aid your observations.

1. Double limb support—Does the pelvic girdle tilt posteriorly to elongate the step length?

     Possible gait deviations:

       excessive or inadequate posterior tilt

2. Single limb support—Does the pelvic girdle tilt anteriorly to promote better axial alignment?

     Possible gait deviations:

       excessive or inadequate anterior tilt

Section B
Pelvic Girdle Motion in the Frontal Plane

Select a member of your lab group to be a walker.

Analyze the pelvic girdle motion in the frontal plane. Place masking tape markers on the walker across both ASIS's and across both PSIS's to assist your visual analysis.

1. Weight acceptance (initial contact and loading response)—Does the pelvic girdle dip slightly to the ipsilateral side?

     Possible gait deviations:

       ipsilateral pelvic drop

       excessive contralateral pelvic drop

       excessive or inadequate pelvic rotation

2. Single limb support—Is the pelvic girdle level in midstance?

     Possible gait deviations:

       ipsilateral pelvic drop

       excessive contralateral pelvic drop

       excessive or inadequate pelvic rotation

3. Preswing—Does the pelvic girdle dip slightly to the contralateral side?

     Possible gait deviations:

       ipsilateral pelvic drop

       excessive contralateral pelvic drop

       excessive or inadequate pelvic rotation

4. Swing phase—Is the pelvic girdle level in midstance?

Does the pelvic girdle rotate forward with swinging limb?

Possible gait deviations:
   ipsilateral pelvic drop
   excessive contralateral pelvic drop
   excessive or inadequate pelvic rotation

Section C
Trunk Motions

Select a member of your lab group to be a walker.

The trunk should remain upright throughout the gait cycle with a slight rotation in the opposite direction of the pelvic girdle. In the sagittal plane, the trunk should be erect with minimal forward or backward leaning. In the frontal plane, observe the space between the upper arms and the chest for symmetry.

The shoulder of the dominant arm may be lower than the nondominant side. Asymmetry may be significantly marked in people engaged in unilateral activities such as baseball pitchers and tennis players.

Possible gait deviations:

   lateral lean to left or right side
   forward or backward lean
   forward or backward trunk rotation
   postural problems such as:
      increased lumbar lordosis
      thoracic kyphosis
      or dorsal scoliosis

Section D
The Arms

Select a member of your lab group to be a walker.

A reciprocal arm swing provides dynamic stabilization of the body and a counterbalance to the swinging limb. An arm swing is not essential for normal gait. People habitually carry, pull, or push objects without demonstrating gait deviations.

   Possible gait deviation:

   abnormal reciprocal swing

Section E
The Head

Select a member of your lab group to be a walker.

As part of the passenger unit, the head should be free to go along for the ride. Head movements should be independent of the torso enabling the eyes and ears to browse the environment and focus on items of interest.

   Possible gait deviations:

   abnormal position or motion

Part 6. Thought Questions

1. Your patient has weak abdominal muscles and a fixed anterior pelvic tilt.

    a. With the patient standing, what compensations would you expect to see at the hip joints and lumbar spine? Explain your answer.

    b. What kind of gait pattern would you expect this patient to exhibit?

2. Your patient has a severe S-shaped scoliotic curve, R thoracic, and L lumbar curves with a pelvic obliquity.

    a. Which pelvis is high?

    b. Describe a gait pattern that you think this patient would most likely exhibit. Explain your answer.

3. You have a patient with a complete lesion of the spinal cord at T_{12}.

    a. List the muscles of the torso that are still functioning.

    b. This patient wants to walk again. Design and describe a gait training program for this patient.

    c. What muscles will this patient use to advance the left extremity during swing phase?

    d. What kind of gait pattern would you recommend for this patient?

    e. Is independent ambulation a reasonable goal for this patient?
       List the factors you would consider when planning a program for this patient.

Part 7. Video Gait Analysis—The Head, Arms, and Torso

Add a new section to your gait form for recording your analysis of HAT kinematics and kinetics. The HAT section should follow the section on the hip in the "O" part of your form. You may want to revise your previous sections to better guide your observations. Use your revised form to analyze the gait of a new walker. Your assignment is to analyze the walker's gait characteristics, foot and ankle function, knee function, hip function, and HAT function in both the sagittal and frontal planes.

In the companion videotape, *People walking: Pathological patterns and normal changes over the life span*, Patient 5 in the first section of the tape can be used for this assignment. His history is as follows.

Walker 5. Age 49

Walker 5 has had multiple sclerosis for 14 years. He uses a straight cane in his left hand and wears a plastic, articulated ankle foot orthosis with a lateral flange on his right leg.

Chapter Six

Gait Through the Life Span

Objectives

1. To discuss some of the motor control theories that influence the acquisition of mature gait.
2. To describe the changing gait patterns seen throughout the life span.
3. To describe variations seen in mature gait patterns as influenced by age, sex, psychological factors, and culture.

Part 1. Terminology

Define the following terms:

1. High guard

2. Primitive patterns

3. Pattern generator

4. Astasia

5. Abasia

6. Reflex

7. Equilibrium reaction

8. Associated movements

9. Cruising

10. Muscle tone

11. Dynamical system

12. Integration

13. Feedback

14. Feed forward

15. Ankle and hip strategies

Part 2. Motor Control Foundations for Mature Gait

Section A
Developmental Reflexes

Reflex hierarchy theories, once held in high regard, have been shown to be oversimplifications. While these theories have been rejected in the light of new research, discussions of developmental reflexes still appear in current literature. Students need to have some familiarity with this material just to be part of the professional conversation. The following section is to acquaint you with some of the developmental reflexes that are associated with gait.

Complete Figure 6-2A-1.

Developmental Reflexes Table				
Reflexes	**Age of Onset**	**Age of Integration**	**Description**	**Significance for Gait**
Prenatal Reflexes				
1. Flexor withdrawal				
2. Crossed extension				
3. Plantar grasp				
4. Neonatal positive supporting reaction				
5. Spontaneous stepping				
6. Proprioceptive placing left extremity (LE)				
Natal and Postnatal Reflexes				
7. Asymmetric tonic neck reflex (ATNR)				
8. Tonic labyrinthine (TLR) reflex—prone and supine				
9. Symmetric tonic neck reflex (STNR)				
Righting Reactions				
10. Labyrinthine head righting				
11. Optical righting				
12. Body on head righting				
13. Mature neck on body righting (NOB)				
14. Mature body on body righting (BOB)				
Equilibrium Reactions				
15. Visual placing LE				
16. Parachute reaction LE				

17. Protective extension upper extremity (UE)
   a. Forward
   b. Sideways
   c. Backwards				

18. Postural fixation in standing				
19. Tilting reaction in standing				
20. Protective staggering				

Figure 6-2A-1.

Section B
Pattern Generator Theories

In contrast to the reflex hierarchy models of motor control are pattern generator theories.

1. Compare and contrast the pattern generator model with the reflex hierarchy model of motor control. In what ways are they similar? In what ways are they different?

2. Explain the ankle and hip strategies described by Nashner (1977, 1979) in the perturbation studies.

3. What is the role of sensory input in the pattern generator model?

4. Critique the pattern generator model. What are the aspects of this model that accurately describe normal movement? What are the aspects of this model that are more problematic? List as many positive and negative aspects as you can.

5. People with neurological deficits exhibit problems in motor control. How would the pattern generator theorists explain the movement problems seen in people with neurological lesions?

Section C
Servomechanism Theory

1. Describe one example of how a closed-loop model could be used to improve a patient's gait.

2. Describe one example of how an open-loop model could be used to improve a patient's gait.

Section D

Dynamical Systems Theory

Thelen, Ulrich, and Jensen (1989) view movement as an interaction between complex, cooperative systems, self-organizing properties, nonlinear dynamics, and phase shifts managed by control parameters. The changes in movement patterns seen during normal infant development can be explained in terms of the dynamics of these systems.

1. Basic concepts

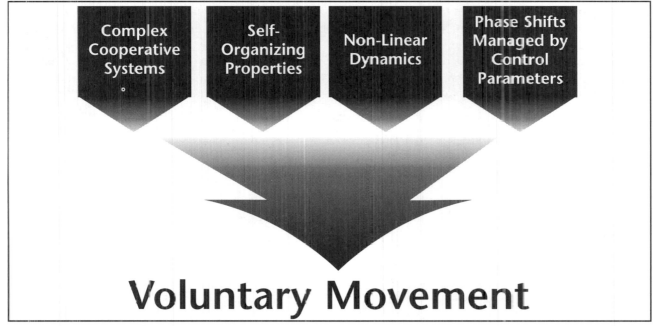

Figure 6-2D-1.

The following activities should help you better understand the dynamical systems model.

a. Complex, cooperative systems

Try this movement experiment—draw several simple shapes on a piece of paper Now try to trace the shapes with a pencil while looking in a mirror instead of at your hand.

What mistakes did you make?

What is the effect of vision on your tracing?

In addition to the sensory and motor systems, list as many systems as you can that influence how we move.

b. Self-organization

This concept means that patterns of movement can develop spontaneously from the interaction of the component systems. Try these movement experiments with the members of your lab group.

i. Have everyone sit facing each other in a circle with both hands in your lap. Now close your eyes and bring one hand to your mouth. Hold it there. Open your eyes and describe the differences in hand placement. Explain the different ways that each person accomplished the task.

ii. Have everyone write his or her name on a piece of paper. Describe the different ways that each person holds the pen or pencil. Try writing your name again. This time change your writing grip to that of another member of your group.

How does it feel to write this new way?

Could you still accomplish the task?

Describe how self-organization enables us to walk at different speeds even though we each have our own preferred "free velocity."

c. Nonlinear dynamics

Try this movement experiment—Take three small objects (hand-sized balls are nice) and juggle them. Let each member of your group try this task.

What are the components necessary for accomplishing this task?

What elements limit a person's ability to juggle three objects?

Could everyone in your group accomplish the task?

Discuss why some people can juggle easily while others cannot.

What contribution did the environment make in accomplishing this task?

List aspects of the environment that made this task easier or harder to accomplish.

During normal motor development, some infants achieve the developmental tasks such as independent sitting and independent creeping sooner than others. Nonlinear dynamics explains that components necessary for accomplishing these tasks mature at different rates. If a necessary component is missing, the task cannot be done. These components are called *rate-limiting* elements. Describe some rate-limiting components in the acquisition of gait.

d. Phase shifts managed by control parameters

Try this movement experiment— Walk slowly along a walkway. Gradually increase your velocity. Continue to increase your velocity until you can no longer maintain a period of double limb support and you are running.

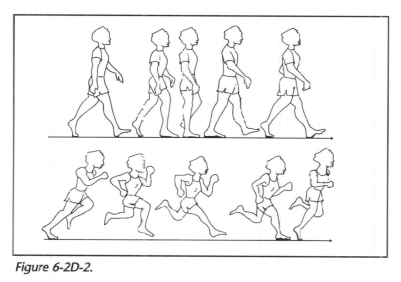

Figure 6-2D-2.

When you switched from fast walking to running, you underwent a phase shift.

What component did you change that finally caused the transition from walking to running?

This component that caused the change in your gait pattern is called a *control parameter*. During normal development, small changes in a few control parameters can cause the transitions that result in independent creeping and independent ambulation.

In your own words, define the term *control parameter* and give some examples.

2. Patterns of movement

Demonstrate the following activities and describe the movement patterns involved. Compare them with the developmental reflexes listed in Part 1. What is the significance of these patterns for gait?

a. You are walking barefoot across a field when suddenly you step on a sharp rock.

b. You are throwing a javelin at the next Olympic games.

c. You are riding on a surfboard and you have just caught the ideal wave.

89

    d. You are waiting in line at a department store cash register when a child runs through the crowd and bumps into you.

3. Joint constraints

A member of your lab group will do the following tasks while the rest of the lab group observes the gait patterns. Time permitting, each member of the lab group should have a turn at being the walker. Note what changes occur in the gait cycle and where they appear. Describe the gait patterns.

    a. Walk wearing a solid ankle-ankle foot orthosis (SA-AFO).

    b. Walk with one foot fixed in maximal ankle plantarflexion.

    c. Walk with one foot fixed in maximal dorsiflexion.

    d. Walk with one foot held in maximal supination.

    e. Walk with one foot held in maximal pronation.

    f. Walk with one knee fixed in at least 30° of flexion.

g. Walk with one knee locked in full extension position.

h. Walk with one hip held in at least 45° of flexion.

i. Walk with both hips maximally internally rotated.

j. Walk with one shoe on and one shoe off.

k. What do joint constraints have to do with the development of normal gait?

4. Postural control

a. Have two members of your lab group walk along a 25-ft walkway. Have the rest of the lab group observe and describe their gait patterns.

Walker 1

Walker 2

b. Now have the walkers close their eyes and have two more members of the group spin them around 10 times. As soon as the spinning is finished, have the walkers again walk along the 25-ft walkway. Describe the changes in the walkers' gait patterns.

Walker 1

Walker 2

c. Describe some of the changes that occur in gait when someone has disturbances in balance and equilibrium.

d. When does the child develop postural control while:
   - prone

   - supine

   - sitting

   - standing

e. What are the implications of the development of balance and equilibrium reactions for acquisition of independent walking?

5. Body constraints

   a. Compare the body proportions of a child with those of an adult. Include in your answer a discussion of relative head size, limb lengths, femoral neck-shaft angles, femoral torsion, tibial torsion, and a ratio of pelvic width to leg length.

   b. Discuss the implications of these different body proportions for the development of normal adult step length, stride length, angle of toe-out, width of base of support (BOS), velocity, and cadence.

6. Muscle strength

    a. Recall some of the gait deviations that resulted from muscle weakness.

    b. Describe why the development of muscle strength, especially extensor muscle strength, is important for the acquisition of independent walking.

7. Motor control

    Thelen et al. (1989) described the following developmental sequence in supine kicking:

        Neonate—Simultaneous activation of flexor and extensor muscles, primarily seen during flexion initiation with extension being relatively passive.

        5 months—Active contractions of flexor and extensor muscles during the appropriate phases of the kick.

        6 to 9 months—Reciprocal coactivation of flexor and extensor muscles.

        7 to 12 months—Selective control of joints is seen.

    Why is selective control of lower extremity muscles necessary for the child to begin to walk?

    If a patient with a neurological lesion cannot achieve selective control of lower extremity muscles but can achieve reciprocal coactivation of flexor and extensor muscles, what kind of gait pattern would this patient demonstrate?

8. Vision

    a. What is meant by the term *optic flow*?

    b. What role does optic flow play in helping infants control their upright posture?

c. Set up a small obstacle course with chairs, cones, or other available objects. Have one member of your group negotiate this course. Now blindfold this person and have him or her walk through the course again. What changes do you see in the person's gait pattern? Time permitting, let each member of your group walk through the course blindfolded and describe the changes that you see in the gait patterns.

9. Psychological factors

a. Motivation is essential for a person to complete a motor task. Thelen et al. (1989) stated that an infant must be able to recognize a goal and desire to achieve it to be able to walk. What motivators do we use in trying to get infants to walk?

b. Gardner (1973) described the stunting of normal growth in children raised in emotionally deprived environments. He found a correlation between emotional stress, environmental deprivation, and hormones secreted by the pituitary gland. These hormones, adrenocortiotrophic hormone and growth hormone, had an inhibitory effect on the emotionally distressed children in his study. Flinn and England (1997) found abnormal levels of salivary cortisol in children living in high stress environments. The abnormal hormone levels in these children corresponded to a diminished immunity and an increase in illnesses. As health professionals, what role can we play in reducing the emotional stress and environmental deprivation of the young patients entrusted to our care?

Part 3. Parental Handling and Influences

Cross-cultural studies link parental handling and attitudes with the onset of independent walking. Reports from the Kipsigis farmers in Kenya (Super, 1976), the !Kung Bushmen of the Kalahari Desert in Botswana (Konner, 1976), and mothers from Jamaica (Hopkins & Westra, 1988) indicate that parental handling can result in earlier independent ambulation. A study from Bali by Mead and Macgregor (1951) showed that parental handling can promote low tone in normal infants and delay independent ambulation.

1. Describe parental handling techniques that increase a child's muscle tone and promote earlier independent walking.

2. Why do you think that Balinese parents in the Mead and Macgregor study wanted their children to have low muscle tone?

3. Mead and Macgregor found that the Balinese children differed from their American counterparts in three major ways: the developmental sequence, habitual movement patterns, and the level of muscle tone. Describe these differences and discuss why they may contribute to a delay in independent walking.

Part 4. Early Gait Patterns

Section A
First Steps

1. Describe the gait pattern of a child who just started independent walking. Include in your answer a description of high-guard and the toddler's gait. (In the companion videotape, *People walking: Pathological patterns and normal changes over the life span*, analyze the gait of the first walker [aged 13½ months] in the developmental sequence to answer this question.)

2. How old were you when you started walking independently?

What is the average age of independent walking for your lab group?

For your class?

For most children in your area?

Discuss reasons for any age differences that you find.

Section B

Gait Patterns in Childhood

Observe normal children walking. Gait characteristics change during normal childhood maturation. Describe the trends of change seen in the following gait characteristics. (In the companion videotape, *People walking: Pathological patterns and normal changes over the life span*, compare the gait of the first two walkers [aged 13½ months and 2 years 7½ months] in the developmental sequence to answer this section.)

    1. Heel strike

    2. Maximal knee flexion during stance

    3. Arm swing

    4. Step length

    5. Stride length

    6. Percentage stance time

7. Single limb support

8. Cadence

9. Velocity

Part 5. Gait and Age

Perry (1992) states that there is a notable decline in people's walking ability after the age of 70 years. Observe the gait of normal adults and describe how the following gait characteristics change as individuals age. (In the companion videotape, *People walking: Pathological patterns and normal changes over the life span*, compare the gait of the last three walkers [aged 23 years, 67 years, and 81 years] in the developmental sequence to answer this section.)

1. Velocity

2. Step length

3. Stride length

4. Width of BOS

5. Angle of toe-out

6. Stance phase

7. Swing phase

8. Double limb support

9. Vertical displacement of center of gravity (COG)

10. Lateral displacement of COG

11. Arm swing

12. Initial contact

13. Joint ranges of motion

14. Joint synchrony

15. Muscle strength

16. Muscle activation patterns

17. Basal metabolic rate

18. Maximal aerobic capacity (VO_2 max)

19. Postural control

20. Sensory input

21. Many characteristics of gait seen in older populations resemble those of the early walker (i.e., reduced step length, reduced velocity, etc.). Discuss this apparent reversal of the developmental process.

Part 6. The Effect of Gender

A number of researchers have shown that men and women walk differently. State the differences you might see between men and women in the following gait variables. Explain your answers.

1. VO_2 max

2. Basal metabolic rate

3. Energy expenditure

4. Step length

5. Stride length

6. Velocity

7. Cadence

Part 7. The Kinesics of Gait

Section A

Age, Sex, and Emotional State

Social scientists report that the way we walk constitutes a form of communication. Birdwhistell (1970) coined the term *kinesics* to describe the nonverbal messages that are conveyed by our movements. Montpare and Zebrowitz (1993) and Montepare and Zebrowitz-McArthur (1988), found that untrained observers could recognize the age, sex, and emotional state of videotaped walkers by characteristics in their gaits.

Lee (1995) reproduced the Montpare and Zebrowitz-McArthur study in Korea and found similar results. What are the gait characteristics that provide untrained observers with clues to the walker's age, sex, and emotional state? Write your hypotheses in the following spaces.

Gait clues to a person's:

1. Age

2. Sex

3. Emotional state

In your lab group, select a walker who will act out the gait of the individuals in the following list. Other members of the lab group will try and guess who the walker is portraying. Lab members will take turns being the walker and demonstrating the different gaits. How do the walkers change their own gait patterns to give a different impression of age, sex, and emotional state?

How good are the observers in guessing the intended age, sex, and emotion?
- *a 20-year-old woman who is very happy*
- *a 25-year-old man who is very angry*
- *a 25-year-old woman who is very tired*
- *a 30-year-old man who is very bored*
- *a 30-year-old woman who is very sexy*
- *a 35-year-old man who is very sexy*
- *a 70-year-old woman who is very tired*
- *a 70-year-old man who is very happy*
- *an 80-year-old woman who is very angry*
- *a 90-year-old man who is very bored*
- *a 90-year-old woman who is very sexy*
- *a 95-year-old man who is very sexy*

Section B
Sociocultural Factors in Gait

Maus (1973) asserted that adult gait patterns arise from cultural conditioning that occurs during childhood. Read the following descriptions of gait and determine who is doing the walking and what is the message that his or her gait patterns convey.

1. "[Their] fac(es) appeared green (i.e., 'pale, depressed'); they walked hunched i[n the street]" (Gruber, 1980).

2. "In general she will walk with her fists closed. And I still can remember my third form teacher shouting at me: Idiot! Why do you walk around the whole time with your hands flapping wide open?" (Maus).

3. "_____ adopted a peculiar gait that was acquired in youth, a loose-jointed swinging of the hips that looks ungainly to us, but was admired by the _____" (Maus).

4. "...with a smile on his grim face, and with his feet below he went with long strides, brandishing his far-shadowing lance" (Bremmer, 1991).

5. "...they resembled in their steps the timorous doves...dainty, delicate, luxurious" (Bremmer).

6. "The little group, stepping silently through the woods, carried bow, arrow, scalping knife, wooden shield and the famous tomahawk..." (Underhill, 1953).

7. "He had a slow, loping walk...only he's imposed on this his own half-beat" (Baldwin, 1965).

Part 8. Thought Questions

1. How important is a knowledge of motor control theories and motor development theories in understanding the acquisition of a normal adult gait pattern? State a position and defend it.

2. Design an ideal early intervention program for children with developmental delays. What kinds of therapeutic interventions would you provide to help them achieve independent walking?

3. How can we distinguish gait changes that occur as a result of the "normal" aging process verses gait changes that result from pathologies?

4. Imagine the gait of a person with hemiplegia or a cerebellar disorder. What nonverbal messages do you think these gaits convey to untrained observers?

5. What do you think of the idea that men and women walk differently? Should physical therapists try and minimize sex differences in the gait patterns of their patients? Discuss your answer.

Chapter Seven

Pathological Gait and Clinical Examples

Objectives

1. To describe the pathological gait patterns seen in clinical cases.
2. To discuss the pathokinematics of gait seen in specific clinical examples.
3. To discuss the pathokinetics of gait seen in specific clinical examples.
4. To discuss the spatial and temporal changes seen in the gait of specific clinical examples.
5. To discuss the motor control problems seen in the gait of specific clinical examples.

Part 1. Spastic Cerebral Palsy—Diplegia and Quadriplegia

Section A
Movement Experiments With Characteristic Gait Patterns

1. Gage (1991) described the characteristic gait pattern of a child with diplegia or quadriplegia as having "flexion, adduction, and internal rotation at the hips and flexion at the knees." Place yourself in this posture.

    a. What is the position of your ankles and feet?

    b. What is the position of your pelvic girdle and dorsal spine?

    Now walk in this posture.

    c. Describe what happens as you shift your weight from one limb to the other.

d. Increase your speed and note any changes that occur in your gait pattern.

2. Perry (1992) called the gait pattern in #1 a *crouch gait*. She added a second pattern involving genu recurvatum. In this pattern, the person with spastic cerebral palsy has flexed hips, hyperextended knees, and plantarflexed ankles. Position yourself so your hips are flexed, your knees are fully extended, and your ankles are plantarflexed.

   a. On what part of your foot are you weight-bearing?
      Describe your base of support (BOS).

   b. What is the position of your pelvic girdle and dorsal spine?

      Now walk in this posture.

   c. Describe what happens as you shift your weight from one limb to the other.

   d. Increase your speed and describe any changes that occur in your gait pattern. Is it easier or harder to walk faster in this gait pattern compared with the crouch gait? Explain your answer.

Section B

Pathokinematics in the Gait of People With Spastic Cerebral Palsy

1. For each of the electric goniometer tracings (Figure 7-1B-1), interpret what is occurring at each joint throughout the gait cycle.

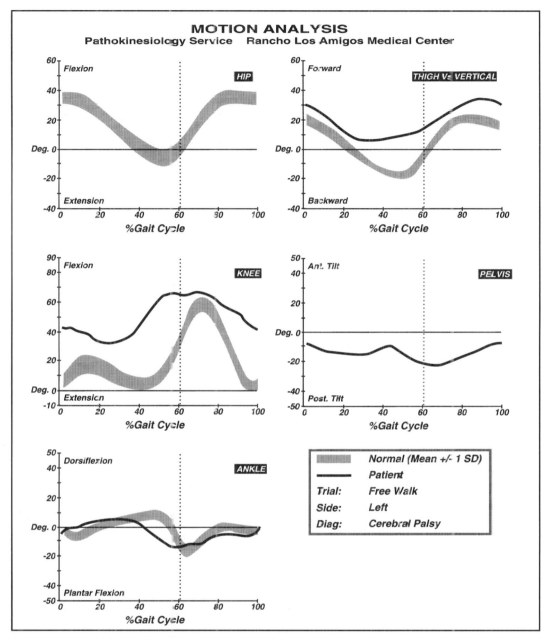

Figure 7-1B-1. Reprinted from Perry (1992).

Ankle

Knee

Hip

Thigh

Pelvis

105

2. Do these tracings illustrate a crouch gait or the genu recurvatum gait pattern?

3. This child has a 5° plantarflexion contracture at the ankle. Can he achieve the 5° dorsiflexion recorded in late midstance?

4. What function does the 5° ankle plantarflexion contracture serve during loading response?

5. This child has a premature heel rise during midstance. What is causing this?

6. This child's thigh exhibits excessive forward positioning during terminal stance. What is causing this?

7. Explain how the thigh can have excessive forward positioning but the hip has nearly normal range of motion (ROM).

Section C
Pathokinetics in the Gait of People With Spastic Cerebral Palsy

1. Look at the dynamic electromyography (EMG) tracings (Figures 7-1C-1 and 7-1C-2). How many gait cycles are represented?

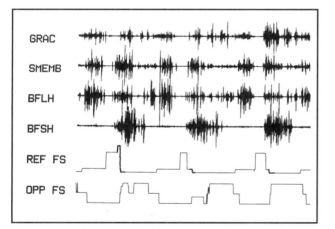

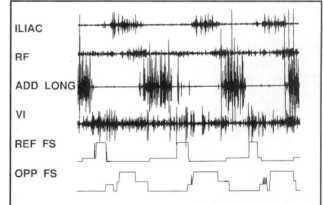

Figure 7-1C-1. Dynamic electromyography, spastic diplegia. GRAC = gracilis; SMEMB = semimembranosis; BFLH = biceps femoris long head; BFSH = biceps femoris short head; REF FS = reference foot switch; OPP FS = opposite foot. Reprinted from Perry (1992).

Figure 7-1C-2. Dynamic electromyography, spastic diplegia. ILIAC = illacus; ADD LONG = adductor longus; RF = rectus femoris; VI = vastus intermedius; REF FS = reference foot switch; OPP FS = opposite foot. Reprinted from Perry (1992).

2. Interpret the muscle activation patterns in Figures 7-1C-1 and 7-1C-2.

3. Compare and contrast the muscle activation patterns of the child with cerebral palsy illustrated in Figures 7-1C-1 and 7-1C-2 and the normal muscle activation patterns seen in Chapters 3 and 4.

Section D

Summarize the main clinical problems seen in this child's gait and suggest a treatment strategy for addressing these problems.

Part 2. Gait of a Person With a Transtibial Amputation

Section A

General Concepts

The goal of lower limb prosthetic management is to give the patient a functional and cosmetically acceptable gait. Despite technological improvements in prosthetic appliances, the gait of people with lower limb amputations still differs from the norm. The following exercises can help you understand why.

1. Sensation

    a. List three types of sensation and explain how each contributes to normal gait.

        i.

        ii.

        iii.

    b. People using lower limb prostheses receive sensory feedback from the artificial limb but not in the same way as a natural limb. Describe three types of sensory feedback patients can get when using a lower limb prosthesis.

        i.

        ii.

        iii.

2. Motion constraints

Few prosthetic joints function as well as natural joints. Some gait abnormalities may be a function of the artificial joint. The most commonly prescribed prosthetic foot in the United States is the nonarticulated solid ankle-cushion heel (SACH) (Shumway-Cook and Woollacott, 1995). It has no moving parts. Foot components include a wooden keel, a polyurethane foam heel wedge and a rubber forefoot. Explain how the SACH foot functions during gait. Include in your answer a discussion of shock absorption, adaptation to uneven surfaces, energy conservation, maintenance of forward momentum, and a comparison of the SACH foot to the natural foot.

3. Postural control

Recall from Chapter 6 the ankle and hip strategies that Nashner and his colleagues (Horak and Nashner, 1986; Nashner, 1977; and Nashner and Woollacott, 1979) described in helping people maintain their upright position during perturbed stance.

Describe the ankle strategy.

Now consider how a person with a lower limb amputation and a prosthetic foot would react to the same perturbation. Describe this reaction and discuss strategies that people with prosthetic legs can use to maintain dynamic equilibrium.

Section B
Pathokinematics

For each of the following electric goniometer tracings (Figure 7-2B-1), interpret what is occurring at each joint throughout the gait cycle.

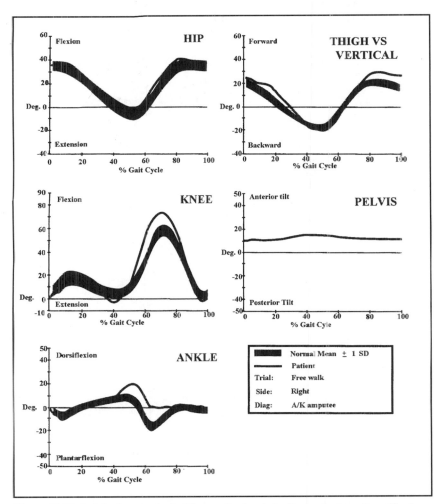

Figure 7-2B-1. Motion analysis. The vertical axis is degrees of motion (flexion is positive). The horizontal axis is the percents of the gait cycle. The vertical dotted line divides stance and swing (toe-off). Gray areas indicate the 1 standard deviation band of normal function. Black line is patient data. Adapted from Perry (1992).

Ankle

Knee

Hip

Thigh

Pelvis

1. What function does the pelvic position play in this person's gait?

2. This person's prosthetic foot permits motion in the sagittal plane. Explain what is happening at the knee when the prosthetic foot has excessive dorsiflexion in terminal stance.

3. Explain why there is a low heel rise and inadequate plantarflexion from preswing through initial swing.

Section C

Pathokinetics

1. Look at the dynamic electromyography tracing (Figure 7-2C-1). How many gait cycles are represented?

2. How would you interpret these muscle activation patterns?

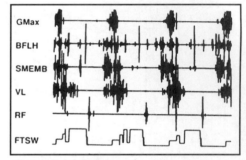

Figure 7-2C-1. Dynamic electromyography. GMax = gluteus maximus; BFLH = biceps femoris long head; SMEMB = semimembranosis; VL = vastus longus (quadriceps); RF = rectus femoris; FTSW = foot switches. Reprinted from Perry (1992).

3. Compare and contrast the muscle activation patterns of this person with the transtibial amputation illustrated in Figure 7-2B-1 and the normal muscle activation patterns seen earlier in Chapters 3 and 4.

Section D

Summarize the main deviations seen in this person's gait and suggest a treatment strategy for addressing these problems.

Part 3. Spinal Cord Injury

Section A

General Concepts

Functional ambulation for people with spinal cord injuries depends on a number of factors. These factors vary from person to person. Hard and fast rules are difficult to formulate and ambulation goals for any particular patient must be set on an individual basis by the treatment team managing the rehabilitation. The following are some of the factors to be considered when setting ambulation goals for a person with a spinal cord injury. For each factor, describe its importance in this goal-setting process.

1. Level of injury—For the levels of spinal cord injury below, list the functional capacities expected for ambulation and explain why.

    a. T_{4-6}

    b. T_{9-12}

    c. L_{1-4}

    d. L_5-S_1

2. Joint contractures

3. Degree of spasticity

4. Body weight

5. Upper body strength, fitness, and general athleticism

6. Sensation

7. Age

8. General health

9. Psychological factors and motivation

10. Sociocultural factors including home and community support systems

Section B

Pathokinematics

The following electric goniometer tracings (Figure 7-3B-1) were made from a person with a spinal cord injury who has regained a community level of ambulation. Interpret what is occurring at each joint throughout the gait cycle.

Ankle

Knee

Hip

Thigh

Pelvis

1. What function does the pelvic position play in this person's gait?

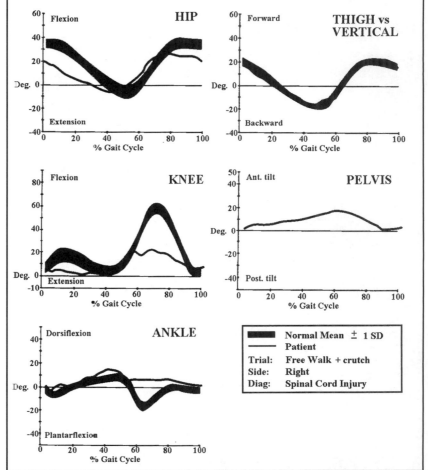

Figure 7-3B-1. Vicon motion analysis. The vertical axis is degrees of motion (flexion is positive). The horizontal axis is the percent of the gait cycle. The vertical dotted line divides stance and swing (toe-off). Gray area indicates the 1 standard deviation band of normal function. Black line is patient data. Adapted from Perry (1992).

2. Which joints display major deviations?
   Give a reason why each deviation is occurring.

3. Analyze what is happening to the right limb during terminal stance. How would this limb pattern affect step length on the left side?

Section C

Pathokinetics

1. Look at the following dynamic EMG tracings (Figures 7-3C-1 and 7-3C-2). Interpret the muscle activation patterns.

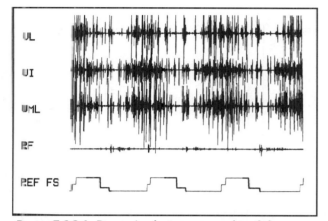

Figure 7-3C-1. Dynamic electromyography of the quadriceps. VML = vastus medialis longus; VI = vastus intermedius; VL = vastus lateralis; RF = rectus femoris; FTSW = foot switches for the reference limb. Reprinted from Perry (1992).

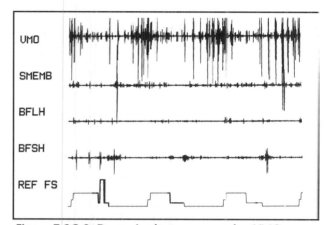

Figure 7-3C-2. Dynamic electromyography. VMO = vastus medialis oblique; SMEMB = semimembranosis; BFLH = biceps femoris long head; BFSH = biceps femoris short head; FTSW = foot switches. Reprinted from Perry (1992).

2. Compare and contrast the muscle activation patterns of this person with a spinal cord injury with the normal muscle activation patterns illustrated earlier in Chapters 3 and 4.

Section D

Summarize the main deviations seen in this person's gait and suggest a treatment strategy for addressing these problems.

Part 4. Peripheral Neuropathy

Section A
General Background

1. Damage to the peripheral nervous system can occur from a number of causes. Give an example of a peripheral neuropathy resulting from the following:

   a. Metabolic disorder

   b. Trauma

   c. Chemical toxicity

2. Complete Figure 7-4A-1 comparing peripheral nerves to upper motor neurons.

Nerve and Neuron Table		
	Peripheral Nerve	**Upper Motor Neuron**
a. Ability to regenerate		
b. Muscle changes after a complete lesion		
c. Sensation when nerve is compressed		
d. Sensation after compression is released		
e. Sensory distribution		

Figure 7-4A-1.

Section B
Pathokinematics

1. Look at the sensory and motor information in Figure 7-4B-1. The patient was a house painter with a long history of using lead-based paints. Explain where in the nervous system the lesion would have to be to produce this clinical picture.

2. Based on the sensory and motor information above, describe the kinematics you would expect to see in this person's gait.

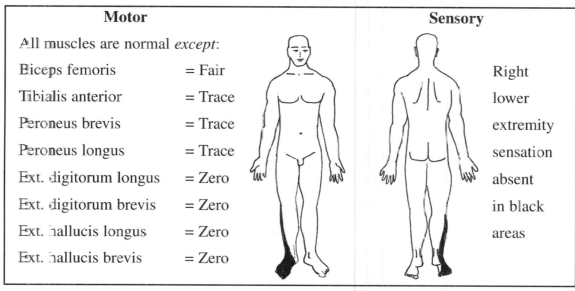

Motor		Sensory
All muscles are normal *except*:		Right
Biceps femoris	= Fair	lower
Tibialis anterior	= Trace	extremity
Peroneus brevis	= Trace	sensation
Peroneus longus	= Trace	absent
Ext. digitorum longus	= Zero	in black
Ext. digitorum brevis	= Zero	areas
Ext. hallucis longus	= Zero	
Ext. hallucis brevis	= Zero	

Figure 7-4B-1. Ext = extensor.

3. Explain how the pathokinematics of this person's gait differ from the kinematics of normal gait.

Section C

Pathokinetics

1. Using the information provided in the sensory and motor charts above, describe the kinetics of this person's gait and explain how this differs from normal gait kinetics.

2. What other motor control issues are relevant to this person's ambulation?

Section D

Summary

Develop goals and a treatment plan for this person.

Part 5. Adult Hemiplegia

Section A
General Concepts

1. Explain why a lesion in the middle cerebral artery can result in hemiplegia.

2. What kind of muscle tone is seen in patients with hemiplegia?

3. The following gait deviations are characteristic of hemiplegic gait. Explain the cause of each gait deviation and describe the gait pattern associated with it.

    a. Drop foot

    b. Genu recurvatum

    c. Excessive hindfoot supination

    d. Inadequate knee flexion

Section B
Pathokinematics

The following electric goniometer tracings (Figure 7-5B-1) were made from a person with hemiplegia. Interpret what is occurring at the ankle and the knee throughout the gait cycle.

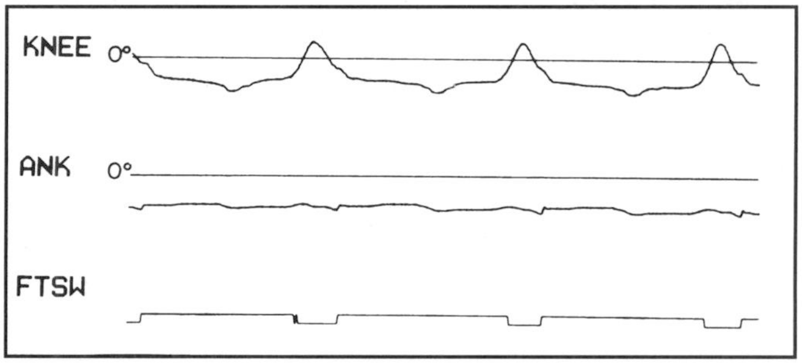

Figure 7-5B-1. Reprinted from Perry (1992).

Ankle

Knee

1. Describe one strategy this patient can use to advance the hemiplegic limb during swing.

2. What kinematics do you expect to see in the hemiplegic hip and pelvis during stance?

3. What kinematics do you expect to see in the contralateral limb during the gait cycle?

Section C

Pathokinetics

1. Look at the following dynamic EMG tracings (Figures 7-5C-1 and 7-5C-2) and interpret the muscle activation patterns.

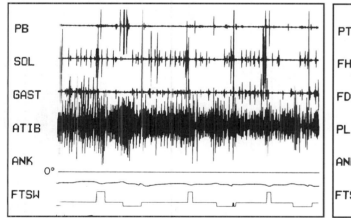

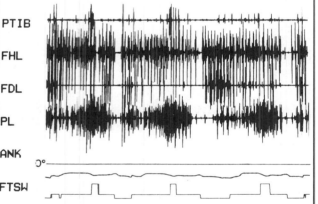

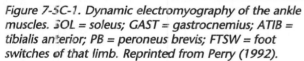

Figure 7-5C-1. Dynamic electromyography of the ankle muscles. SOL = soleus; GAST = gastrocnemius; ATIB = tibialis anterior; PB = peroneus brevis; FTSW = foot switches of that limb. Reprinted from Perry (1992).

Figure 7-5C-2. Dynamic electromyography of the perimalleolar muscles. PTIB = posterior tibialis; FHL = flexor hallucis longus; FDL = flexor digitorum longus; PL = peroneus longus. Reprinted from Perry (1992).

2. Compare and contrast the muscle activation patterns of this person with hemiplegia with the normal muscle activation patterns seen earlier in Chapters 3 and 4. Describe this comparison.

Section D

Summarize the main deviations seen in this person's gait and suggest a treatment strategy for addressing these problems.

Part 6. Gait Deviations in People With Parkinson's Disease

1. Where in the nervous system is the lesion producing the clinical picture of Parkinson's disease? Be as specific as possible.

2. List the characteristic signs and symptoms of Parkinson's disease.

3. Describe the characteristic gait associated with Parkinson's disease.

4. In general, what are the ankle, knee, and hip joint kinematics you would expect to see in the gait of someone with Parkinson's disease?

5. In general, what kind of muscle activation patterns would you expect to see in the gait of someone with Parkinson's disease?

6. Summarize the main gait deviations seen in people with Parkinson's disease and suggest a treatment strategy for addressing these problems.

Part 7. Gait Deviations in People With Down Syndrome

1. Down syndrome is a genetic disorder. Describe three ways that Down syndrome can occur.

2. Describe the general clinical signs and symptoms of Down syndrome.

3. Describe the gait typically seen in people with Down syndrome.

4. List some of the kinematic factors characteristic of Down syndrome gait.

5. List some of the kinetic factors characteristic of Down syndrome gait.

6. Summarize the main gait deviations seen in people with Down syndrome and suggest a treatment strategy for addressing these problems.

Part 8. Center of Gravity Displacement Problems

Section A
General Concepts

To maintain a static upright posture, the body must be able to arrange its body parts to keep its body's COG over its base of support. Displacement of COG will either cause the body to fall or necessitate some sort of postural adjustment to accommodate the displacement. Try the following movement experiments:

Choose a member of your lab group to be the model. The model will stand in a relaxed posture with both hands at the side. The model will do the activities listed below and the other members of the lab group will record the postural changes that occur with the motion. After each activity the model will resume the original relaxed standing position.

1. Flex the right hip to 60°.
2. Flex the trunk at the waist as far as possible, bringing both arms forward.
3. Flex both knees as far as possible without moving at the hip joints.
4. Dorsiflex at both ankles as far as possible.
5. Summarize the observations and make a general statement about postural adjustments to COG displacement.

Section B
Center of Gravity Displacement and Postural Compensations—Sagittal Plane

1. Recall the COG displacement that occurs during gait.
   a. List as many mechanisms as you can recall that control vertical COG displacement.

   b. List as many mechanisms as you can recall that control lateral COG displacement.

2. Recall a contractile and a noncontractile problem for each body region listed in the Figure 7-8B-1 that causes the ground reaction force vector to be displaced *anteriorly* and describe a compensation for this problem that is seen during gait.

Anterior Contractile/Noncontractile Problem Table		
	Problem	**Compensation**
a. Foot and Ankle		
contractile		
noncontractile		
b. Knee		
contractile		
noncontractile		
c. Hip		
contractile		
noncontractile		
d. Pelvic girdle		
contractile		
noncontractile		
e. Dorsal spinal		
contractile		
noncontractile		

Figure 7-8B-1.

3. Recall a contractile and a noncontractile problem for each body region listed in the Figure 7-8B-2 that causes the ground reaction force vector to be displaced *posteriorly* and describe a compensation for this problem that is seen during gait.

Posterior Contractile/Noncontractile Problem Table		
	Problem	**Compensation**
a. Foot and Ankle		
contractile		
noncontractile		
b. Knee		
contractile		
noncontractile		
c. Hip		
contractile		
noncontractile		
d. Pelvic girdle		
contractile		
noncontractile		
e. Dorsal spinal		
contractile		
noncontractile		

Figure 7-8B-2.

Section C

Center of Gravity Displacement and Postural Compensations—Frontal Plane

1. Recall a contractile and a noncontractile problem for each body region listed in Figure 7-8C-1 that causes the ground reaction force vector to be displaced laterally and describe a compensation for this problem that is seen during gait.

Frontal Plane Compensation Table		
	Problem	**Compensation**
a. Foot and Ankle		
contractile		
noncontractile		
b. Knee		
contractile		
noncontractile		
c. Hip		
contractile		
noncontractile		
d. Pelvic girdle		
contractile		
noncontractile		
e. Dorsal spinal		
contractile		
noncontractile		

Figure 7-8C-1.

2. Formulate a general rule that will help you distinguish clinical problems from postural compensations in your observational gait analysis.

Answer
Key

Answer Key

Chapter 1
Part 1. Terminology and Basic Concepts
Section A

1. Gait cycle—all of the activities that occur starting with a specific event on one foot until that event is repeated on the same foot. Some people measure the gait cycle from heel contact on one foot to the next heel contact of the same foot. Other people measure the gait cycle from toe off on one foot to the next toe off of the same foot.

2. Stance phase—one of two phases of the gait cycle. It begins when the reference foot contacts the floor and ends when the reference foot lifts off the ground. In normal adults, stance phase begins with initial heel contact and ends with the toe coming off the ground. Stance phase is 60% of the normal adult gait cycle.

3. Swing phase—second of two phases of the gait cycle. It begins when the reference foot lifts off the ground and ends when the reference foot contacts the floor. In normal adults swing phase is 40% of the gait cycle.

4. Single limb support—that part of the gait cycle when only one foot is in contact with the ground. In normal adults, single limb support constitutes 80% of the gait cycle and occurs when one limb is in midstance and terminal stance and the opposite limb is in swing phase.

5. Double limb support—that part of the gait cycle when both feet are in contact with the ground. In normal adults, single limb support constitutes 20% of the gait cycle and occurs during loading response at the beginning of stance phase and preswing at the end of stance phase.

6. Stride length—a linear distance measured along the line of progression representing how far the body has traveled in one gait cycle. Usually measured from the posterior aspect of one heel to the posterior aspect of the same heel during two successive floor contacts. Values for normal adults are as follows: average for women: 4.2 f or 1.28 m, average for men: 4.8 ft or 1.46 m, overall average: 4.6 ft or 1.41 m.

7. Step length—a linear distance measured along the line of progression representing how far one foot has traveled during a gait cycle. Usually measured from the posterior aspect of one heel to the posterior aspect of the opposite heel during two successive floor contacts. The length of two steps equals a stride. Values for normal adults are as follows: average for women: 2.1 ft or 0.64 m, average for men: 2.4 ft or 0.73 m, overall average: 2.3 ft or 0.705 m.

8. Cadence—the number of steps taken in a specified amount of time. Usually measured as the number of steps per second or the number of steps per minute. Values for normal adults are as follows: average for women: 117 steps/min, average for men: 111 steps/min, overall average: 113 steps/min.

9. Walking velocity—the speed of ambulation on a smooth level surface; values for normal adults are as follows: Average for women: 250 ft/min or 77 m/min, average for men: 276 ft/min or 86 m/min, overall average: 262 ft/min or 82 m/min.

10. Width of base of support (BOS)—a linear distance measured perpendicular to the line of progression from the center of the posterior aspect of one heel to the center of the posterior aspect of the opposite heel. Values for normal adults are 2 to 4 inches or 5.08 cm to 10.16 cm.

11. Angle of toe-out—Angle formed by the line of progression and the longitudinal axis of the foot. Normal adults have about 7° of toe-out.

12. HAT—Term introduced by Elftman (1954) to describe the head, arms, trunk, and pelvic girdle: also called the passenger unit.

13. Ground reaction force vector (GRFV)—the sum of three forces acting on the body is equal and opposite to the amount of momentum generated by the foot and the body during stance phase; the three forces include a vertical force, an anterior-posterior force and a lateral force. The GRFV is useful for people trying to understand gait because it helps them visualize muscle contractions and other kinematic factors needed to control the body's joints during locomotion.

14. Center of gravity (COG)—point in a body around which all of the forces act; in a human body standing in the anatomical position, the COG is approximately just anterior to sacral level 2. Answer Figure 1-1A-2 shows the center of gravity with an X on sacral 2 level.

15. Center of pressure (COP)—a point on a body's supporting surface around which all of the forces act; during gait, COP is measured on the plantar aspect of the walker's feet. Answer Figure 1-1A-3 shows the line of pressure.

Section B

A   Double limb support

B. Single limb support

C. Angle of toe-out

D. Width of BOS

E. Step length

F. Stride length

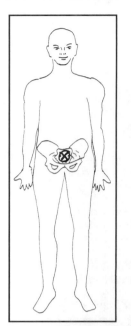

Answer Figure 1-1A-2.

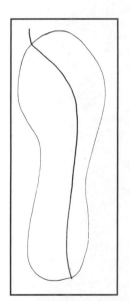

Answer Figure 1-1A-3.

Section C

The Gait Cycle Terminology

Answers to Figure 1-1C-1.
1. A. IC.
   B. LR.
   C. MSt.
   D. TSt.
   E. PSw.
   F. ISw.
   G. MSw.
   H. TSw.

2. Subdivisions of the gait cycle.

Stance Phase					
	1	*2*	*3*	*4*	*5*
RLA	IC	LR	MSt	TSt	PSw
Traditional	HS	FF	MSt	HO	TO
% of GC	0%-2%	0%-10%	10%-30%	30%-50%	50%-60%
Swing Phase					
	1	*2*	*3*		
RLA	ISw	MSw	TSw		
Traditional	AC	MSw	DC		
% of GC	60%-73%	73%-85%	85%-100%		

Answer Figure 1-1C-3. GC = gait cycle.

Section D

Basic Functions

The Passenger Unit

1. COG for the HAT is just anterior to the tenth thoracic vertebra (T_{10}).

2. This arrangement makes static posture very difficult because stability is dependent on good alignment of the body parts. The top-heavy nature of the passenger unit is inherently unstable.

   Dynamic locomotion is possible only if the person can control the moving body parts. Walking can be regarded as a controlled fall from one limb to the other.

The Locomotor Unit

3. The eleven joints are: lumbosacral, both hips, knees, ankles, subtalars, and metatarsalphalangeal joints.

4. Pelvic girdle: it is the base of the passenger unit and the most superior component of the locomotor unit.

The Ground Reaction Force Vector

5. GRFV promotes stable alignment when the COG is aligned over the BOS. Torque is generated when the COG of the body part moves beyond the BOS.

6. The body's COG and the COP on the stance foot.

Quiet Standing

7. Body weight, ligamentous tension, and muscle activity.

8. Hip, hyperextension; knee, extension; ankle, dorsiflexion.

9. Posterior to the hip, anterior to the knee, and slightly anterior to the ankle.

10. Both joints are in their close-packed positions.

11. The ankle is not in its close-packed position. The body tends to sway and muscle power is necessary to control this.

12. Toe-out is approximately 7°, which serves to widen the BOS.

Dynamic Stability

13. On the average: 3.5 inches when standing and 3 inches when walking.

14. During quiet standing we do not have the benefit of inertia and forward momentum, which provide additional stabilization during gait, so a greater BOS is necessary.

15. Our COG shifts 1 inch to each side for a total of 2 inches. The average walking BOS is 3 inches. Inertia and forward momentum assisted by muscle contractions prevent us from falling over.

Normal Gait and Kinetics

16. Stance phase kinematics and kinetics.

Joint	IC	LR	MSt	TSt	PSw
Hip					
Motion	flexion 30°-25°	flexion 30°-25°	extension	extension	flexion
GRFV	anterior	anterior	anterior→posterior	posterior	posterior→0
Moment	flexion	flexion	little→0	extension	extension
Muscle group	gluteus maximus, hamstrings, addus magnus	gluteus maximus, hamstrings,	quiet	addus longus in late TSt	flexors
Contraction	isometric	isometric	quiet	eccentric	concentric
Knee					
Motion	flexion 5°	flexion	extension	extension→flexion	flexion
GRFV	anterior	posterior	posterior→anterior	anterior→posterior	posterior→0
Moment	extension	flexion	flexion→extension	extension→flexion	flexion→0
Muscle group	quadriceps, hamstrings, popliteus	quadriceps	quadriceps→0	gastrocnemius popliteus	gastrocnemius popliteus
Contraction	eccentric (quadriceps) concentric (hamstrings)	eccentric	concentric→0	eccentric →concentric	concentric
Ankle					
Motion	plantarflexion 0°	plantarflexion	dorsiflexion	dorsiflexion→ plantarflexion	plantarflexion
GRFV	posterior	posterior	anterior	anterior	anterior
Moment	plantarflexion	plantarflexion	dorsiflexion	dorsiflexion	dorsiflexion→0
Muscle group	dorsiflexors	dorsiflexors	plantarflexors	plantarflexors	plantarflexors
Contraction	eccentric	eccentric	eccentric	eccentric→ concentric	concentric

Answer Figure 1-1D-3. IC = initial contact; LR = loading response; MSt = midstance; TSt = terminal stance; PSw = preswing; GRFV = ground reaction force vector.

17. Swing phase kinematics and kinetics.

Joint	ISw	MSw	TSw
Hip			
Motion	flexion	flexion	flexion, extension at end
Muscle group	flexors	addus longus, gracilis	extensors
Contraction	concentric	concentric	eccentric
Knee			
Motion	flexion	extension	extension→flexion
Muscle group	hamstrings, sartorius, gracilis	hamstrings	hamstrings, quadriceps, popliteus
Contraction	concentric	eccentric	eccectric→concentric
Ankle			
Motion	dorsiflexion	dorsiflexion	dorsiflexion
Muscle group	dorsiflexors	dorsiflexors	dorsiflexors
Contraction	concentric	concentric	isometric/concentric

Answer Figure 1-1D-4. ISw - initial swing; MSw = midswing; TSw = terminal swing.

Forward Progression

18. Rocker systems showing the effort arm (EA), resistance arm (RA), and vector forces.

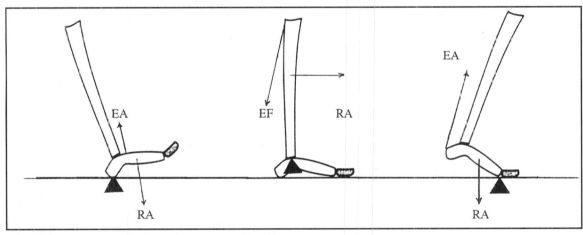

Answer Figure 1-1D-5. Adapted from Perry (1992).

a. Heel rocker   b. Ankle rocker   c. Forefoot rocker

19.

a. Forefoot rocker—the body's weight is at the end of a long lever arm (the stance limb). Dorsiflexion during terminal stance places the GRFV over the metatarsal heads increasing the dorsiflexion moment at the ankle. The metatarsal heads serve as a fulcrum for the forefoot rocker and the body falls forward contributing to forward momentum of the limb.

b. Rapid unloading of the body's weight onto the contralateral limb—the contralateral limb is in front of the passenger unit. Inertia, assisted by the adductor muscles, directs the body weight forward and laterally. The trailing limb follows the body.

c. Knee flexion—concentric contraction of the triceps surae plantarflexes the ankle and flexes the knee. Knee flexion results in tibial advancement.

d. Hip flexor action—concentric contraction of the hip flexor muscles advances the femur and contributes to knee flexion and tibial advancement.

20. Hip flexion during initial swing brings the trailing limb forward and upward, contributing more force to the passenger unit and **131**

conserving forward momentum and inertia.

21. Knee extension in late swing maintains the forward advancement of the thigh and the shin by continuing the momentum of the distal segments of the limb. This momentum (like the old "Crack-the-Whip" game) provides a pulling force on the body and adds to the force generated by the body's weight falling forward over the stance limb.

Shock Absorption

22. Ankle plantarflexion—the swinging limb comes to an abrupt halt as the heel contacts the ground. Ankle plantarflexion enables some of this limb to continue moving, conserving some inertia. The pretibial muscles eccentrically lower the foot to the floor, restraining plantarflexion, and slowing foot flat. This muscle action reduces some of the force generated by initial impact.

23. Subtalar pronation—the initial contact occurs on the lateral aspect of the calcaneus. The ground reaction forces push the calcaneus laterally, resulting in pronation at the subtalar joint. The hindfoot and the midfoot pronate in rapid succession entering their loose-packed positions, permitting accessory motion and enabling shock absorption in all of the joints of the foot.

24. Knee flexion—as the pretibial muscles act to restrain rapid ankle plantarflexion, they pull on the shin. With the calcaneus as the fulcrum of the heel rocker, the entire ankle-foot-shin complex is pitched forward. This action causes the anterior displacement of the knee's anatomical axis with respect to the GRFV and increases the flexion moment at the knee. To control the flexion moment, the vasti eccentrically contract and absorb some of the shock generated by initial impact.

25. Hip flexion—the hip is held in approximately 25° to 30° of flexion during most of the loading response. The GRFV is anterior to the hip joint and a flexor moment is present. The hip extensor muscles control the flexor moment and absorb some of the shock of impact.

26. Hip abductors—as the stance limb begins to accept the weight from the contralateral limb, the pelvis drops to the contralateral side. This drop is controlled eccentrically by the hip abductors of the stance limb enabling these muscles to also participate in shock absorption.

Energy Conservation

27. a. Two inch total; 1 inch up and 1 inch down.

   b. Midstance.

   c. Lateral and anterior tilt of the pelvis, ankle plantarflexion, and knee flexion.

   d. Double limb support.

   e. Terminal stance heel rise, initial heel contact with knee extended, horizontal pelvic rotation.

28. a. Two inch total; 1 inch to each side.

   b. Midstance.

   c. Pelvic rotations, medial femoral angulation, inertia negating the necessity for the body's COG to be balanced over the stance foot (see #15 in Section D).

29. Whenever possible, the body substitutes passive positioning, inertia, and momentum for muscle action. Muscle contractions occur selectively during stance phase, mostly to eccentrically control moments generated around the GRFV. The timing and intensity of muscle activity is modulated by the serial demand of torques passing from the hip at initial contact to the knee during loading response through the ankle at terminal stance. This selective activation of muscles minimizes energy expenditure.

Part 2. Activities

Answers depend on individual lab groups.

Part 3. Thought Questions

1. Pelvic rotation narrows the BOS and minimizes lateral COG displacement.

2. Normal pelvic motions minimize vertical COG displacement. Abnormal pelvic motions may increase it.

3. a. Displaces the COG anteriorly: to maintain balance, a compensatory posterior COG displacement must occur somewhere else in the closed chain.

   b. Knee flexion contractures cause an increased demand on the quadriceps. If the quadriceps are not strong enough to meet this demand, the body may accommodate by shifting the GRFV anterior with respect to the knee. This shift lessens the flexion moment and decreases the demand on the quadriceps. Two ways to accomplish this are forward trunk flexion or an anterior pelvic tilt.

   c. A plantarflexion contracture interferes with the heel and the ankle rockers. The body has a problem with terminal stance heel rise and initial heel contact with the knee extended when ankle motion mediates the COG from falling too low and at mid-stance when ankle alignment with knee flexion controls the COG from rising too high. A variety of strategies are seen clinically to compensate plantarflexion contractures. Some of these strategies include vaulting over the contracture which results in an excessive vertical displacement of the COG, recurvatum at the knee resulting in a backward displacement of COG, or excessive knee flexion which causes an increased demand on the quadriceps muscle and may result in the clinical picture described in answer b.

   d. Increased vertical displacement of the COG.

   e. Pelvic girdle instability and a compensation displacing the COG laterally either toward or away from the involved side.

   f. A narrowing of the width of BOS; trunk lateral flexion may increase to the left to raise the pelvic girdle and substitute for hip abduction. This will increase COG displacement to the left side.

4. If velocity stays the same, step length and stride length will decrease. If step length and stride length stay the same, velocity will increase.

5. Your COG displacement may or may not change but the mechanisms that conserve forward momentum will not be as effective and you will have a more energy-demanding gait.

6. Yes, gait characteristics will change because pelvic motions will be restricted. Step length, stride length, and velocity may all be decreased. Width of BOS, cadence, and lateral COG displacement can all be expected to increase.

7. *Errors in validity*: many answers are possible; here are a few. Angle of observation, poor or distracting lighting, estimation of measurements, lack of measuring scale for comparisons, lack of observer's experience doing a gait analysis, and lack of patient cooperation.

   Errors in reliability: many answers are possible; here are a few. Doing the gait analysis at different times of the day, in different places and under different conditions, patient fatigue, lack of observer's experience doing a gait analysis, lack of patient cooperation, multiple inexperienced observers, and estimation of measurements.

8. *Minimizing errors in validity*: many answers are possible; here are a few. Observe the walker at 90° to the plane of motion (in the sagittal and frontal planes), observe the walker in a well-lit room with a minimal amount of distractions. Use measurements instead of estimations, a reference scale, and gain as much experience as possible in gait analysis. Explain the procedure to the walker ahead of time so as to gain his or her maximal amount of cooperation.

   Minimizing errors in reliability: many answers are possible; here are a few. Do repeated gait analyses in the same room, at the same time of day, and under the same conditions. Use observers who have a high level of experience doing gait analyses, videotape walkers at 90° to plane of motion (in the sagittal and frontal planes) to minimize walker fatigue. Use the same reference scale for all gait analyses, minimize the use of estimations, and maximize the use of direct measurements.

9. Pelvic rotation in the transverse plane functionally elongates the limbs during double limb support by rotating forward and adding pelvic width to the length of the step. The pelvis also tilts posteriorly during double limb support and this also functionally elongates the limbs and effectively lengthens the step.

10. Pelvic rotation, terminal stance heel rise, initial heel contact with knee extended, medial femoral angulation, and inertia negate the necessity for the body's COG to be balanced over the stance foot.

11. Decreased proprioception and decreased kinesthesia will make it hard for the walker to know where the impaired limb is in space. Walkers may damage or overstretch joints without realizing it. Lack of pain sensation may result in skin damage because walkers will not notice that their shoes or orthotic appliances are abrading the skin.

12. a. 30° flexion.

    b. 30° to 45° flexion.

    c. 15° plantarflexion.

    d. A feedback mechanism designed to prevent destruction of the joint by excessive pressures inhibits muscle contractions.

13. Spasticity: increased muscle tone resulting from an upper motor neuron lesion.
Clonus: rapid, alternating muscle contractions of agonists and antagonists due to a hyperactive stretch reflex resulting from an upper motor neuron lesion.

14. a. People with neurological lesions who have a decreased ability to adapt to postural demands may have difficulty maintaining their balance during gait. These people may show fixed stereotypical patterns of movement, a loss of flexibility, changes in the gait parameters (a wider BOS, a slower velocity, shorter or uneven step lengths, etc.), and an inability to adapt to uneven surfaces.

    b. People with central nervous system lesions often demonstrate a lack of selective muscle activation. This means both an inability to recruit muscles during their normal activation period and the inability to inhibit abnormal muscle contractions occurring during periods when these muscles are normally quiet. Limb movements appear stiff, stereotypical, and lacking the mechanisms that promote shock absorption, energy conservation, and forward progression. People with spasticity may demonstrate persistent activation of gastrocsoleus resulting in excessive plantarflexion and the loss of the ankle rocker. Hamstring spasticity may result in excessive knee flexion during terminal stance and decreased thigh advancement during swing. A variety of other gait deviations are also seen clinically.

    c. The term "primitive pattern" refers to limb patterns that are seen normally during infancy. Two of these patterns are the total limb flexion and extension patterns seen as part of the positive (extension, weight bearing) and negative (flexion, nonweight bearing) supporting reactions of the extremities. These patterns are seen in people with spastic disorders in both the affected upper and lower extremities.

15. *Ataxia:* usually seen in a person with a lesion in the cerebellum or in a cerebellar pathway. An ataxic gait has a wide BOS, incoordination with delays in the initiation of movement, or errors in the range, force, or rhythms of movement.

Hemiplegia: usually seen in people with lesions in the internal capsule or a lesion in the middle cerebral artery. Hemiplegic gait affects the upper extremity and lower extremity on the same side of the body. Muscle tone is usually abnormal and may range from low to absent (completely flaccid) to extremely high (severely spastic). Muscle weakness is also a problem. During gait, primitive patterns are seen in both affected extremities.

During periods of increased effort, the affected upper extremity may demonstrate a flexion pattern with a clenched fist. The affected lower extremity may demonstrate an extension pattern during stance phase and a flexion pattern during swing phase. Variations of these patterns include a drop foot (excessive plantarflexion) during swing, genu recurvatum during single limb support, and a stiff-knee gait throughout the cycle.

Festination: seen in people with Parkinson's disease, with lesions in the basal ganglia's substantia nigra. Parkinsonian gait involves a rigid, flexed trunk; nonswinging, forward flexed arms; flexion at the hips and knees; and short, shuffling steps that increase in cadence as if the feet are trying to catch up to the displaced forward COG.

Chapter 2
Normal and Pathological Foot and Ankle Function
Part 1. Terminology

(Many answers can be found in the literature. Here are some examples.)

Section A

Functional Parts of the Foot

1. Hindfoot—calcaneus and talus.

2. Rearfoot—calcaneus and talus.

3. Midfoot—three cuneiforms, navicular, and cuboid.

4. Forefoot—anterior aspect of the foot: composed of the metatarsals and phalanges.

5. Ray—a functional unit composed of the metatarsals and their associated cuneiform bones.

6. Longitudinal arch—functional complex of bones composed of the hindfoot, midfoot, and metatarsals.

Section B

Motions of the Foot and Ankle

1. Dorsiflexion—motion of the foot in the sagittal plane around a frontal-transverse axis such that the distal segment of the foot approaches the shin.

2. Plantarflexion—motion of the foot in the sagittal plane around a frontal-transverse axis such that the distal segment of the foot moves away from the shin.

3. Inversion—motion of the foot in the frontal plane around a sagittal-transverse axis such that the plantar aspect of the foot moves toward the midline of the body.

4. Eversion—motion of the foot in the frontal plane around a sagittal-transverse axis such that the plantar aspect of the foot moves away from the midline of the body.

5. Adduction—motion of the foot in the transverse plane around a sagittal-frontal axis such that the distal aspect of the foot moves toward the midline.

6. Abduction—motion of the foot in the transverse plane around a sagittal-frontal axis such that the distal aspect of the foot moves away from the midline.

7. Supination—a triplanar motion of the foot around an oblique axis involving a combination of the following three motions: adduction, inversion, and plantarflexion.

8. Pronation—a triplanar motion of the foot around an oblique axis involving a combination of the following three motions: abduction, eversion, and dorsiflexion.

Section C

Deformities of the Foot and Ankle

1. Equinus—a sagittal plane deformity of the foot in which the foot is fixed in plantarflexion.

2. Calcaneovarus—a deformity of the foot in which the ankle joint is fixed in dorsiflexion and the foot is fixed in inversion.

3. Pes cavus—a sagittal plane deformity resulting in an abnormally high longitudinal arch.

4. Pes planus—a sagittal plane deformity resulting in an abnormally low longitudinal arch; also used for feet fixed in pronation.

5. Talipes calcaneus—a sagittal plane deformity of the foot in which the ankle joint is fixed in dorsiflexion.

6. Hindfoot varus—a frontal plane deformity of the foot in which the calcaneus is deviated toward the midline and the plantar aspect of the foot is turned medially.

7. Hindfoot valgus—a frontal plane deformity of the foot in which the calcaneus is deviated away from the midline and the plantar aspect of the foot is turned laterally.

8. Forefoot varus—a frontal plane deformity of the foot in which the metatarsals are deviated toward the midline.

9. Forefoot valgus—a frontal plane deformity of the foot in which the metatarsals are deviated away from the midline.

10. Hallux abductovalgus (HAV)—a deformity involving all three planes: the midfoot hyperpronates resulting in a collapse of the medial longitudinal arch and a medial rotation of the first ray. In this new position, the long flexor muscles of the hallux pull the big toe laterally when they contract.

Part 2. Normal Functional Anatomy

Section A

Osteology

Location of the bones and joints of the foot.

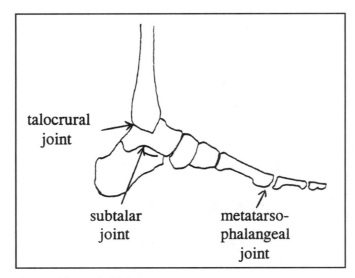

Answer Figure 2-2A-1.

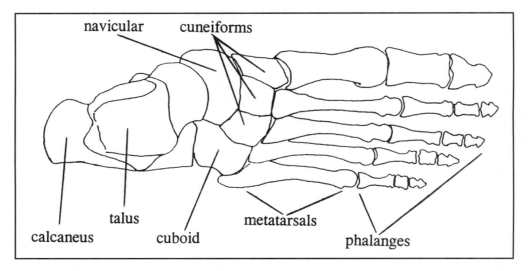

Answer Figure 2-2A-2.

Section B

Arthrology

The Talocrural Joint

1. The talocrural joint axis is only 11° off from being aligned with the transverse-frontal axis. Movement around the talocrural joint axis is technically supination and pronation because the axis is oblique. We normally call motion at the talocrural joint dorsiflexion and plantarflexion because these motions predominate.

2. Dorsiflexion.

3. More limitation of plantarflexion than dorsiflexion with a hard end-feel.

4. 15°.

The Subtalar Joint

1. Supination and pronation.

2. Supination.

3. A and B have more articular surface than the other variations and so have the possibility of more joint motion. D and E have the least amount of articular surface and have joint geometries that restrict motion. D and E represent hypomobile joints.

4. Open chain: foot supination is related to shin external rotation; foot pronation is related to shin internal rotation.

   Closed chain: foot supination is related to shin external rotation; foot pronation is related to shin internal rotation.

   A mitered hinge is a metal joint connecting two side pieces that are oriented 90° to each other. The axis joint of the hinge is oriented 45° to the long axis of each side piece. This arrangement results in each side piece moving in its own unique plane.

5. In the paper model of the mitered hinge, increases in the axis angle resulted in decreased foot motion and increased shin motion. One study found this to be true in human cadaver feet (Bruckner 1987) but a second study found that the relationship was more complex and a direct correlation could not be made (Baker et al., 1992). The knee has a moving axis of rotation. The knee functions like a modified hinge joint. The femoral condyles glide and roll on the tibial plateau. If the subtalar joint has a single stationary axis then this joint is relatively simple to treat orthotically or simulate prosthetically. If the subtalar joint has a single moving axis or multiple axes of rotation then the motion is more complex and more difficult to treat if there is a dysfunction.

Section C

The Arches of the Foot

1. A medial longitudinal arch lowers from initial contact (IC) through loading response (LR) and raises from midstance (MSt) through preswing (PSw).

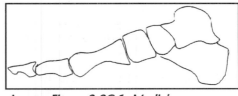

Answer Figure 2-2C-1. Medial longitudinal arch.

2. A lateral longitudinal arch remains stable and rigid throughout the gait cycle.

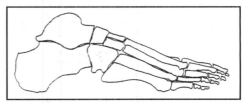

Answer Figure 2-2C-2. Lateral longitudinal arch.

3. A transverse arch lowers from IC through LR and raises from MSt through PSw; the proximal aspect of the transverse arch participates in the peroneal pulley mechanism and the distal aspect of the transverse arch assists in distributing the body weight between the metatarsal heads.

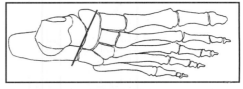

Answer Figure 2-2C-3. Transverse arch.

4. The medial longitudinal arch lowers during foot pronation.

5. The medial longitudinal arch rises during foot supination.

6. The lateral longitudinal arch remains stationary during stance phase.

7. The ligaments and the plantar aponeurosis bind the structures of the foot together so they function like an arch or a beam. When the foot pronates and the joints of the hindfoot and midfoot enter their loose-packed positions, the ligaments and the plantar fascia loosen, permitting accessory joint motion to absorb the shock of initial contact and loading response. When the hindfoot and the midfoot supinate, the ligaments and the plantar fascia become taut, the medial longitudinal arch rises and the foot becomes a rigid structure capable of withstanding the forces encountered during single limb support.

8. If the longitudinal arches do not serve their intended function, problems can arise. One problem is hyperpronation. If the medial longitudinal arch collapses medially, hyperpronation results. The foot remains pronated in late stance and the joints are in their loose-packed positions. Loose-packed joints cannot play their role in raising the foot's longitudinal arch or in accommodating the increased vertical forces that accompany heel rise and the forefoot rocker. Plantar fascia and the intrinsic structures of the foot also support the foot's longitudinal arch but they are not designed to handle the increased ground reaction forces of terminal stance without support from the bones and joints. Without this support, the plantar fascia can tear, resulting in plantar fasciitis. Repeated trauma to the plantar fascia at its osseous attachment on the calcaneus can produce a heel spur.

9. The peroneus longus tendon runs through the groove on the cuboid and under the cuneiform bones to insert on the lateral side of the base of the first metatarsal and medial cuneiform bone. Peroneus longus is active from early MSt through the end of terminal stance (TSt). The open chain action of peroneus longus is foot pronation. This muscle is contracting during stance phase while the foot is supinating. During gait, the peroneus longus contracts eccentrically to bind the cuboid and cuneiform bones together, stabilize the transverse arch, and support the rising medial longitudinal arch.

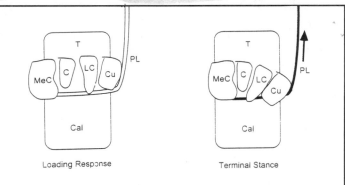

Answer Figure 2-2C-4.

Part 3. Normal
Foot and Ankle Function—Sagittal Plane

Section A

Kinematics

Curve describing movement of the ankle joint.

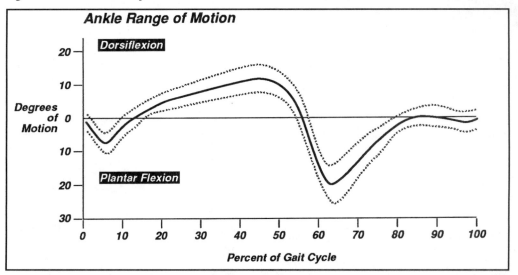

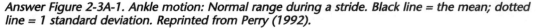

Answer Figure 2-3A-1. Ankle motion: Normal range during a stride. Black line = the mean; dotted line = 1 standard deviation. Reprinted from Perry (1992).

Section B

Kinetics

Answers to Figure 2-3B-1:
The muscles in consecutive order are: tibialis anterior, extensor hallus longus, extensor digitorum longus.

Answers to Figure 2-3B-2: soleus, gastrocnemius, posterior tibialis, flexor digitorum longus, peroneus brevis, peroneus longus.

Gait Subdivision Table	
1. Maximal dorsiflexion (ROM)	TSt - heel off
2. Maximal plantarflexion (ROM)	ISw - accel.
3. Ankle dorsiflexor activity (MMT)	LR, PSw, ISw, MSw, TSw
4. Ankle plantarflexor activity (MMT)	MSt, TSt

Answer Figure 2-3B-3. TSt = terminal stance; ISw = initial swing; LR = loading response; PSw = preswing; MSw = midswing; TSw = terminal swing; MSt = midstance.

To understand the relationship between the position of the ankle and the activation of specific muscle groups, look at the ground reaction force vector (GRFV), identify the moment, and determine which muscles can counteract this moment.

Part 4. Normal Foot and Ankle Function—Frontal Plane

Section A

Kinematics

Curve describing movement of the subtalar joint.

Answer Figure 2-4A-1.

Section B

Kinetics

1. Peronei, extensor digitorum longus, and some slight help from extensor hallus longus.

2. The plantarflexor muscles (because of their attachment on the calcaneus), tibialis posterior, and some contributions from tibialis anterior and flexor hallus longus.

3. LR.

4. PSw.

5. Muscles are working eccentrically.

Part 5. Pathomechanics of the Foot

Section A

Pathomechanics—Excessive Ankle Plantarflexion

1. Points in the cycle for gait deviations.

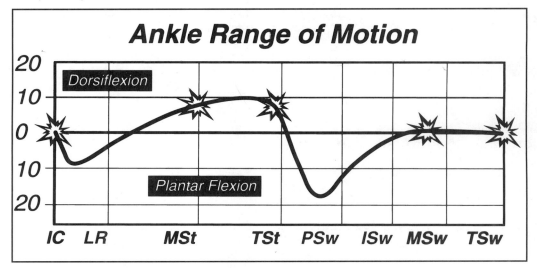

Answer Figure 2-5A-1. Reprinted from Perry (1992).

2. Many answers are possible. Here are three:

   a. Hot, painful joint 2° rheumatoid arthritis—the position of most comfort and least intra-articular pressure is 15° plantarflexion. Possible gait deviations include: shortened step on painful side, slower velocity to decrease GRFV, low heel strike or footflat contact, absent or decreased heel and ankle rocker, early heel rise in MSt, forward trunk lean, shortened step contralateral side, excessive hip and knee flexion with possible lateral trunk lean to clear the toes, excessive plantarflexion in terminal swing (TSw).

   b. Joint contracture—possible gait deviations include: shortened step on contracted side, slower velocity to decrease GRFV, low heel strike or footflat contact, absent or decreased heel and ankle rocker, early heel rise in MSt, genu recurvatum during single limb support, forward trunk lean, shortened step on contralateral side, toe drag, excessive hip and knee flexion with possible lateral trunk lean to clear the toes, excessive plantarflexion in TSw.

   c. Lateral ankle sprain—possible gait deviations include: shortened step length and time on painful side, slower velocity to decrease GRFV, low heel strike or footflat contact, absent or decreased heel and ankle rocker, early heel rise in MSt, forward trunk lean, excessive hip and knee flexion with possible lateral trunk lean to clear the toes, excessive plantarflexion in TSw.

3. a. Spasticity of the gastrocsoleus muscle—depending on the severity of the spasticity, the triceps surae may be active throughout the gait cycle or activated in TSw to function as part of the extensor pattern that enables weight-bearing during stance phase. During PSw, the person initiates a flexion pattern that involves hip and knee flexion and ankle dorsiflexion. This flexion pattern enables the foot to be lifted off the ground and swing phase to begin. The activation of the ankle dorsiflexors

inhibits the triceps surae and activation of the gastrocsoleus may decrease or cease during initial swing (ISw) and midswing (MSw).

    b. Weakness of tibialis anterior—the ankle dorsiflexors are active from IC through LR to eccentrically lower the foot to the floor and during swing phase to enable foot clearance.

4. Excessive plantarflexion during stance uses the closed chain effect to extend the knee, displace the GRFV anteriorly, and protect a weak quadriceps muscle from injury. Excessive plantarflexion during LR reduces the heel rocker mechanism and lessens the forces causing tibial advancement. Knee extension is maintained and the GRFV is displaced anteriorly stabilizing the knee and minimizing the need for strong quadriceps. This strategy begins in TSw with soleus activation causing ankle plantarflexion and tibialis anterior controlling the rate. A low heel strike occurs at IC and a rapid footflat occurs during LR. Calf muscle activity restrains tibial advancement and, using the closed chain mechanism, continues knee extension. Forward progression of the tibia is controlled by the calf muscles through MSt and TSt. Maximal ankle dorsiflexion is seen late in PSw instead of TSt resulting in prolonged heel contact and continued knee extension.

Section B

Pathomechanics—Excessive Ankle Dorsiflexion

1. During swing, excessive dorsiflexion helps with foot clearance and does not disrupt the forward progression of the limb. In stance, excessive dorsiflexion in IC exaggerates the heel rocker and destabilizes the knee. Throughout stance phase, excessive dorsiflexion will increase the forces causing tibial advancement, increase knee flexion, and place a greater demand on the quadriceps.

2. Pattern A describes a sudden dorsiflexion of the ankle after the ankle plantarflexes during LR. Ankle dorsiflexion is maintained through stance until the end of TSt.

3. Pattern B describes a progressive increase in ankle dorsiflexion from MSt through TSt.

4. a Joint contracture—adhesions in the joint holding it in dorsiflexion.

    b Talipes calcaneus—a foot deformity that fixes the ankle in dorsiflexion.

    c Excessive knee flexion—positions the ankle in excessive dorsiflexion to achieve footflat.

5. a. Soleus weakness from disuse, paralysis, or the result of a poor surgical outcome from an Achilles tendon lengthening. Weak plantarflexors cannot control the tibia during stance resulting in excessive dorsiflexion.

    b. Primitive flexion patterns seen in patients with neurological lesions may show excessive dorsiflexion during swing when the entire limb pattern is activated.

6. Gait deviations would include an obstruction of the heel rocker because plantarflexion is not permitted. Footflat is achieved by a rapid advance of the tibia causing increased knee flexion, increased quadriceps demand, and a destabilized knee. In MSt, the ankle rocker is not possible because the orthotic ankle joint is fixed in neutral. Forward progression of the tibia is achieved by increasing the demand on the forefoot rocker. In late stance, the entire shin-foot complex proceeds forward as a unit, resulting in an early heel rise, increased tibial advancement, increased quadriceps demand and an unstable knee.

7. Increased knee flexion.

Section C

Foot Deformities and Gait Deviations—Sagittal Plane

1. Pes cavus—gait deviations follow the pattern seen with excessive plantarflexion; low heel contact during IC; early footflat seen during LR. In MSt the tibia may have difficulties with forward advancement necessitating some compensation at the knee (such as excessive extension) or at the foot (such as hyperpronation or excessive supination). The rest of the gait cycle may not be affected.

2. Equinus—gait deviations follow the pattern seen with excessive plantarflexion; low heel or forefoot contact seen during IC; early footflat seen during LR. In MSt the tibia may have difficulties with the ankle rocker mechanism and forward advancement necessitating some compensation at the knee (such as excessive extension or excessive flexion) or at the foot (such as hyperpronation); early heel rise may occur in late MSt; problems with foot clearance may be seen during swing.

3. Talipes calcaneus—gait deviations follow the pattern seen with excessive dorsiflexion; excessive heel rocker at IC. In LR there is increased tibial advancement, increased knee flexion, increased quadriceps demand, and an unstable knee. In MSt and TSt

there is a continuation of increased tibial advancement, increased knee flexion, increased quadriceps demand, and a prolonged heel contact. In PSw, prolonged heel contact continues and normal plantarflexion is lost. A significant problem seen during swing is the position of the ankle (excessive dorsiflexion) at the end of TSw in preparation for the next IC.

4. Pes planus—IC may look normal. The foot may excessively pronate during LR and remain pronated throughout stance phase. A low heel rise or prolonged heel contact may be seen in TSt. In PSw, prolonged heel contact may continue and normal plantarflexion is reduced.

Section D

Foot Deformities and Gait Deviations—Frontal Plane

1. Hindfoot varus—at IC the foot contacts the ground on the lateral aspect of the heel. The foot hyperpronates during LR to achieve foot flat. Hyperpronation is seen through MSt and TSt but resolves as the heel rises. A medial heel whip may occur with heel rise and the foot returns to its normal alignment as it rises and weight is shifted to the opposite limb.

2. Forefoot varus—IC looks normal. Hindfoot and midfoot hyperpronation begins during LR with forefoot contact and continues throughout stance.

3. Forefoot valgus—IC looks normal but the hindfoot and midfoot show decreased pronation during LR and an increased amount of supination from MSt through TSt. As the heel rises, the hindfoot pronates and may even exhibit a lateral heel whip. Hindfoot and midfoot pronation may continue through PSw until the foot lifts off the ground.

Section E

Foot Deformities and Gait Deviations—Triplanar

1. Equinovarus—combination of the gait deviations seen with an equinus deformity and a hindfoot varus deformity.

2. Forefoot supinatus—the forefoot is in a fixed position of plantarflexion, adduction and inversion. IC and LR will look fairly normal, excessive pronation will be seen during single limb support and resolve only after toe-off.

3. Hindfoot varus with forefoot supinatus—the foot begins to pronate at IC and remains in excessive pronation throughout the stance phase.

4. Hyperpronation—usually refers to hyperpronation through the transverse tarsal joint. Gait deviation looks like the hyperpronation variation seen with hindfoot varus.

5. Hallux abductovalgus (HAV)—a deformity resulting from midfoot hyperpronation and usually hindfoot varus. At IC weight is accepted on the lateral aspect of the heel. Excessive pronation occurs during LR and persists through TSt. This excessive pronation causes the medial longitudinal arch to drop and the first ray to rotate medially. The long flexor muscles of the hallux pull the big toe into abduction and during PSw and the foot lifts off on the medial aspect of the hallux.

Section F

Gait Deviations

Answers to Figure 2-5F-1.

1. Foot slap—seen during IC through LR, caused by very weak or absent dorsiflexors. Significance: poor heel rocker, decreased shock absorption, and decreased forward progression.

2. Forefoot or footflat contact—seen during LR, caused by plantarflexion contracture, weak dorsiflexor muscles, spastic or contracted plantarflexor muscles, compensation for weak quadriceps muscles, and heel pain. Significance: poor heel rocker and decreased forward progression, and decreased shock absorption by decreasing knee flexion.

3. Excessive dorsiflexion—seen during IC through LR, caused by talipes calcaneus, dorsiflexion contracture of the ankle joint, poor surgical outcome of Achilles tendon lengthening, and compensation for excessive hip and knee flexion. Significance: increased heel rocker and forward progression, increased demand on quadriceps, destabilizing effect on the limb; during MSt and TSt. Weak plantarflexors, forefoot pain, compensation for inadequate hip and knee extension. Significance: increased demand on quadriceps, interferes with heel rise, and serves to decrease step length of contralateral limb.

4. Delayed heel contact—seen during LR, caused by plantarflexion contracture, spastic or contracted plantarflexor muscles, and equinus deformity. Significance: poor heel rocker and decreased forward progression.

5. Premature heel rise—seen during MSt, caused by plantarflexion contracture, spastic or contracted plantarflexor muscles, and equinus deformity. Significance: increased forward advancement of the shin, increased flexion of the knee, and increased demand on the quadriceps.

6. Prolonged heel contact (or delayed heel rise)—seen during PSw, caused by talipes calcaneus, excessive dorsiflexion, and weak plantarflexor muscles. Significance: increased demand on the quadriceps and decreased step length of the contralateral limb.

7. Hyperpronation—seen from IC to LR through TSt, caused by a hindfoot varus deformity with ligamentous laxity of the midfoot. The foot does not become a rigid structure (close-packed in hindfoot and midfoot) and cannot meet the demands of the increased ground reaction forces of TSt, which may result in hallux abductovalgus. Seen from TSt through PSw, caused by a forefoot varus deformity. Significance: lateral heel whip, poor forefoot rocker, and poor progression over forefoot. Seen from LR through PSw, caused by a forefoot varus. Significance: poor forefoot rocker and poor progression over forefoot. Seen throughout stance phase, caused by a hindfoot varus with forefoot supinatus. Significance: may result in valgus strain at the knee, foot pain, and poor forward progression.

8. Excessive hindfoot supination—seen throughout the stance phase, caused by equinovarus deformity, plantarflexion contracture, weak peroneals, tibialis anterior and posterior spasticity, soleus spasticity, and motor control problems in the hindfoot. Significance: poor positioning for IC, decreased shock absorption, and decreased stability during single limb support.

9. Medial heel whip—seen from heel off through PSw, caused by a forefoot varus or forefoot supinatus deformity and may be increased if patient has increased muscle tone. Significance: increased torsion force on metatarsal heads and poor forefoot rocker.

10. Lateral heel whip—seen from heel off through PSw, caused by a forefoot valgus and may be increased if patient has increased muscle tone. Significance: increased torsion force on metatarsal heads and poor forefoot rocker.

11. Foot or toe drag—seen during swing phase, caused by weak dorsiflexors, uncompensated plantarflexion contracture, inadequate flexion at the hip or knee, and motor control problems; impaired proprioception. Significance: interferes with limb advancement and may compromise balance.

12. No heel off—seen during TSt and PSw, caused by weak plantarflexors, forefoot pain, a compensation for excessive ankle dorsiflexion, or inadequate toe extension. Significance: interferes with forefoot rocker and forward progression, decreases step length of contralateral limb, and may result in inadequate knee flexion during swing phase.

13. Vaulting over contralateral limb—seen during swing phase, caused by short stance limb or relatively too long swing limb, and compensation for decreased knee flexion, or plantarflexion contracture of swing limb. Significance: increased demand on plantarflexors on stance limb.

14. Increased toe extension—seen during swing phase, caused by toe extensors substituting for lack of foot clearance of swing limb. Lack of clearance may be caused by a weak tibialis anterior, a plantarflexion contraction at the ankle, inadequate knee flexion, inadequate hip flexion, or a long swing limb. Significance: may assist with foot clearance, or may cause calluses or skin irritation of toes rubbing on the inside of the shoe.

15. Claw toes—seen during MSt and TSt, caused by increased muscle tone, plantar grasp reflex, muscle imbalance of toe extensors and flexors, and a compensation for a weak soleus. Significance: interferes with ankle rocker and forward progression, and decreases step length of contralateral limb.

Section G

Sensory Factors

1. Peripheral nerve lesion (i.e., peroneal nerve), spinal cord injury, central nervous system lesion, lesion in skin resulting in decreased or absent receptors.

2. Decreased kinesthesia, decreased proprioception, substituting visual placing of the feet for normal postural reactions, substituting auditory clues for proprioception input (i.e., foot slap), bruises, calluses, and blisters from unperceived irritations caused by shoes, orthotic or prosthetic appliances, or by direct trauma.

3. Claw toe during stance, excessive toe-up during swing, the primitive extension pattern seen during stance and the primitive flexion pattern seen during swing, sustained muscle activity due to hypersensitivity to slow stretch.

4. a. The patient wants to avoid weight-bearing on the painful limb so he or she shortens step length (e.g., a sprained ankle, a blister caused by a shoe rubbing on the Achilles tendon).

b. The patient reduces intra-articular pressure; pain inhibits the muscles from acting so joint pressures are minimized (e.g., a joint with rheumatoid arthritis).

c. Reflexively inhibiting muscle activation (e.g., in the case of a fracture, pain inhibits the muscle from contracting).

Section H

Motor Control Deficits

1. Spasticity and clonus—jerky or tremulous movements occur during gait and the movements do not look smooth, graceful, or normal. Problems in postural control and dynamic balance arise as patients have difficulty initiating movement and maintaining a smooth progression through the gait cycle. The rocker mechanisms are compromised and eccentric muscle contractions are obstructed.

2. Lack of selective muscle control—difficulty seen in activating individual muscle groups and in controlling the rate, magnitude, and timing of muscle contractions. Distal control is affected more than proximal control.

3. Primitive locomotor patterns—patients with neurological lesions exhibit limb patterns seen in infants who have just started independent ambulation. During stance, patients display the extension synergies seen in positive supporting reactions. During swing, patients demonstrate flexion patterns seen in negative supporting reactions. These patterns substitute for voluntary control.

4. Inappropriate phasing of muscle activation—spastic muscles demonstrate inappropriate phasing. Their contractions may be too late, too early, too long, continuous, or absent.

5. Sensory deficits and inadequate sensory feedback makes it difficult for the walker to know where the involved limb is in space or to protect the joints from injury. Patients may have difficulty placing the limb during early stance, stabilizing the limb during single limb support, and shifting body weight to the opposite limb at the end of stance. Patients with plantarflexor spasticity or quadriceps weakness can stand on a knee in extreme hyperextension without severe complaints of pain or even recognition of the situation. Problems in sequencing the gait pattern may indicate processing errors in addition to sensory deficits.

Part 6. Observational Gait Analysis—The Foot and Ankle

Answers depend on individual lab groups.

Part 7. Thought Questions

Section A

1. Hallux abductovalgus can result from hindfoot varus and hyperpronation. During IC through LR, the foot contacts the ground on the lateral aspect of the heel and hyperpronates to achieve foot flat. Hyperpronation collapses the medial longitudinal arch medially. During MSt and TSt, the foot is loose-packed when it needs to be close-packed. The foot does not become a rigid structure (close-packed in hindfoot and midfoot) and cannot meet the demands of the increased ground reaction forces of TSt. When the long toe extensors try to contract while the medial longitudinal arch is collapsed and medially rotated, their line of action is laterally deviated and the muscles of the big toe end up pulling it into abductovalgus.

2. On the long side during stance, the patient's center of gravity may be dramatically displaced vertically. During swing phase, the short limb may vault to clear the long side. Look for compensations that would functionally elongate the short side (excessive ankle plantarflexion, decreased knee flexion, decreased hip extension) or functionally shorten the long side (excessive hip abduction throughout stance phase, decreased ankle plantarflexion, increased knee flexion or increased hip flexion). The patient could also have unequal step lengths and step times.

3. A windlass is a winch used on a boat to hoist or haul objects. The windlass has been used as a model to explain how hyperextension at the metatarsal phalangeal joints can pull on the plantar aponeurosis and increase a cavus deformity. Because the plantar aponeurosis is attached to the phalanges any dorsiflexion at the metatarsalphalangeal joints will increase tension in the plantar structures. The situation becomes more aggravated if the patient has claw toes and a pes cavus. Now any dorsiflexion at the metatarsalphalangeal joints pulls the tight planar aponeurosis even tighter and further exacerbates the cavus deformity.

4. Answers to Figure 2-7A-1. Delayed heel contact (LR)—caused by excessive plantarflexion. Seen in patients with plantarflexion contractures, soleus spasticity, weakness or paralysis of tibialis anterior, and primitive extension patterns.

Answers to Figure 2-7A-2. Premature heel off (MSt)—caused by excessive plantarflexion. Seen in patients with plantarflexion contractures, soleus spasticity, weakness or paralysis of tibialis anterior, and primitive extension patterns.

Answers to Figure 2-7A-3. Prolonged heel contact (TSt and PSw)—may be caused by soleus weakness, excessive dorsiflexion, or excessive plantarflexion with genu recurvatum causing problems in forward progression and limb advancement.

Chapter 3
Normal and Pathological Knee Function
Part 1. Terminology

Section A

Motions of the Knee

1. Flexion—sagittal plane motion around an axis at the intersections of the frontal and transverse planes in which the distal aspects of both segments come closer together.

2. Extension—sagittal plane motion around an axis at the intersections of the frontal and transverse planes in which the distal aspects of both segments move farther apart.

3. Internal or medial rotation—transverse plane motion around an axis at the intersections of the sagittal and frontal planes in which the segments rotate toward the midline.

4. External or lateral rotation—transverse plane motion around an axis at the intersections of the sagittal and frontal planes in which the segments rotate away from the midline.

5. Adduction—frontal plane motion around an axis at the intersections of the sagittal and transverse planes in which the distal segment moves toward the body's midline.

6. Abduction—frontal plane motion around an axis at the intersections of the sagittal and transverse planes in which the distal segment moves away from the body's midline.

Section B

Deformities of the Knee

1. Genu varus—frontal plane deformity in which the knee is fixed in a position of adduction.

2. Genu valgum—frontal plane deformity in which the knee is fixed in a position of abduction.

3. Genu recurvatum—sagittal plane deformity in which the knee hyperextends beyond the normal limits.

4. Patella alta—an abnormally high patella, may present with a "camel's sign" (lateral view of knee shows two "humps": one for the high-riding patella and one for the exposed infrapatella fat pad).

5. Osgood-Schlatter disease—enlargement of the tibial tubercle.

Part 2. Normal Functional Anatomy

Section A

Osteology

Answers to Figure 3-2A-1.

1.A. Medial tibial plateau. B. Lateral tibial plateau. C. Medial femoral condyle. D. Lateral femoral condyle. E. Intercondylar tubercles. F. Fibular head.

2. Full extension.

3. Enables internal rotation, external rotation, and gliding of the femoral condyles on the tibial plateau.

4. The *screw home* mechanism enables the knee to lock in full extension. In the final degrees of knee extension, the femur rotates medially on the tibia until it achieves full extension and its close-packed or locked position. This mechanism is not normally

seen during stance phase but can be used pathologically as a strategy for bearing weight on an unstable knee.

5. The patella is the largest sesamoid bone in the body and functions to increase the mechanical advantage of the quadriceps muscle. The patella alters the direction of quadriceps action, changing the moment arm, and increasing the amount of torque that can be generated.

6. The physiological valgus at the knee seen in adults enables the width of base of support to be narrower than the width of the pelvis. During gait, the narrower base helps conserve energy because lateral displacement of the center of gravity (COG) is minimized.

Section B

Arthrology

1. Capsular pattern: greater limitation of flexion than extension; both rotations free.

2. a. The menisci function to enhance articular congruency of femoral condyles with the tibial plateau, distribute weight-bearing forces, absorb shock, and reduce friction.

   b. The anterior cruciate ligament functions to restrain anterior displacement of the tibia with respect to the femoral condyles.

   c. The posterior cruciate ligament functions to restrain the posterior displacement of the tibia with respect to the femoral condyles.

   d. The medial collateral ligament functions to resist valgus stress (abduction) and restrains excessive lateral rotation of the tibia. It is most effective when the knee is slightly flexed.

   e. The lateral collateral ligament functions to resist varus stress (adduction) and restrains excessive lateral rotation of the tibia with posterior displacement. It is most effective when the knee is slightly flexed.

   f. The coronary ligaments bind the menisci to the tibial plateau.

Section C

Osteokinematics and Arthrokinematics

1. In full extension, the femur is medially rotated and locked in position. The popliteus contracts to laterally rotate the femur with respect to the tibia and initiate flexion. The femoral condyles slide anteriorly and roll posteriorly as flexion continues. The joint axis moves in a small arc posteriorly and superiorly until full flexion is achieved.

Diagram showing movement of the femur on the tibia.

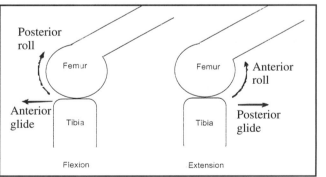

Answer Figure 3-2C-1. Reprinted from Perry (1992).

2. a. During flexion, the femur slides anteriorly and rolls posteriorly.

   b. During extension, the femur slides posteriorly and rolls anteriorly.

3. a. The femur rotates laterally when the knee is flexing.

   b. The femur rotates medially when the knee is extending, especially at the end of range.

4. a. The knee adducts during flexion.

    b. The knee abducts during extension.

Part 3. Normal Knee Function—Sagittal Plane

Section A

Kinematics

Movement of the knee joint during the gait cycle.

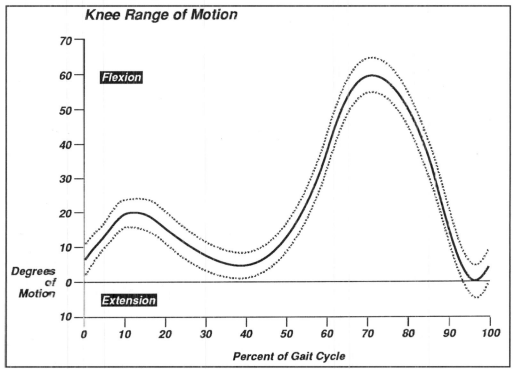

Answer Figure 3-3A-1. Reprinted from Perry (1992).

Section 3

Kinetics

Answers to Figure 3-3B-1: The muscles in consecutive order are: knee flexors: biceps femoris (short head), popliteus, gastrocnemius.

Answers to Figure 3-3B-2: gracilis and sartorius.

Answers to Figure 3-3B-3: biceps femoris (long head), semimembranosis, semitendonosis.

Answers to Figure 3-3B-4: knee extensors: vastus intermedius, vastus lateralis, vastus medialis longus, vastus medialis obliquus, rectus femoris.

Gait Subdivision Table	
1. Maximal knee flexion (ROM)	ISw
2. Maximal knee extension (ROM)	TSw
3. Extensor muscle activity (MMT)	IC, LR and early MSt, TSw
4. Flexor muscle activity (MMT)	Some knee flexors are always working during the gait cycle

Answer Figure 3-3B-5. ROM = range of motion; ISw = initial swing; TSw = terminal swing; MMT = manual muscle test; IC = initial contact; LR = loading response; MSt = midstance; TSw = terminal swing.

147

Muscles are active to oppose the ground reaction forces. When the ground reaction force vector (GRFV) is anterior to the knee joint, an extension moment occurs and is controlled by flexor muscles. When the GRFV is posterior to the joint a flexion moment occurs. During loading response (LR), the flexor moment is controlled by the knee extensor muscles. During preswing (PSw), the flexor moment decreases to zero as the foot comes off the ground so control of the ground reaction forces is not necessary.

Part 4. Normal Knee Function—Transverse Plane

Internal rotation of the limb occurs from initial contact (IC) through LR. As the body enters single limb support, external rotation begins and continues through the end of stance phase. As the foot comes off the ground, the limb again starts internally rotating. This rotation will continue through LR of the next gait cycle. The biceps femoris muscle passively helps control tibial internal rotation.

Part 5. Knee Function—Frontal Plane

1 Knee abduction begins at IC, increases slightly during LR and is maintained during stance phase.

2. Knee adduction occurs during swing and increases with knee flexion.

3. The iliotibial band provides a lateral restraint of adduction torque.

Part 6. Knee Pathomechanics

Section A

Kinematics

Parts of the gait cycle where abnormal knee function is significant.

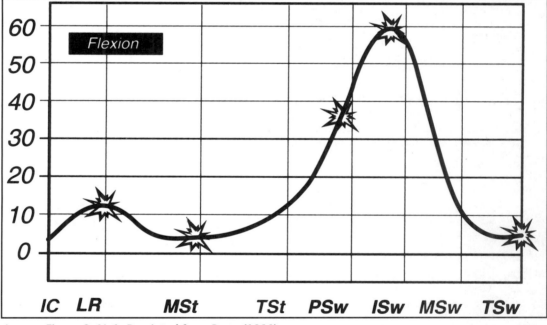

Answer Figure 3-6A-1. Reprinted from Perry (1992).

Section B

Specific gait deviations

A. Inadequate flexion

1. Descriptions of unilateral and bilateral inadequate flexion should include gait deviations that occur during LR, PSw, and initial swing (ISw). Many variations of gait deviations are possible.

2. During LR, knee flexion functions to absorb shock, enabling the heel rocker mechanism to operate smoothly, and slowing down the upward vertical displacement of COG from double limb support to single limb support.

During PSw and ISw, knee flexion functions to facilitate the forefoot rocker, enabling thigh advancement, assisting with foot clearance, and combining with the hip flexors in bringing the trailing limb closer to the body.

3. Noncontractile reasons for inadequate knee flexion include: joint contracture, knee pain secondary to arthritis (flexion restricted mostly PSw and ISw), peroneal nerve problems (deviation seen during LR), or primitive extension pattern (deviation seen during weight-bearing).

4. A. Contractile reasons for inadequate knee flexion include: quadriceps weakness, quadriceps spasticity, hip flexor weakness, soleus contracture (deviation seen during LR), or ankle plantarflexion spasticity (deviation seen during LR).

B. Excessive extension and extensor thrust

1. Extensor thrust involves a quick extension of the knee that locks it in its close-packed position and enables weight-bearing.

2. Extensor thrust can be caused by quadriceps weakness, an ankle plantarflexion contracture, or ankle plantarflexion spasticity.

Descriptions of the gait deviations vary depending on the compensations employed by the walkers.

C. Hyperextension

1. Hyperextension can be caused actively by quadriceps spasticity, ankle plantarflexion spasticity, or a primitive extension pattern.

2. Passive causes for knee hyperextension include laxity of posterior joint structures, quadriceps weakness, an ankle plantarflexion contracture, or a cavus or equinus foot deformity.

D. Excessive flexion

1. Descriptions of the gait deviations vary depending on the compensations employed by the walkers.

2. Causes of excessive knee flexion include: hamstring spasticity, knee flexion contracture, hip flexion contracture, ankle dorsi flexion weakness, ankle dorsiflexion spasticity, or a peroneal nerve lesion.

E. Inadequate extension

1. Descriptions of the gait deviations vary depending on the compensations employed by the walkers.

2. Causes of inadequate knee extension include: hamstring spasticity, knee flexion contracture, hip flexion contracture, ankle plantarflexion weakness, or a primitive flexion pattern seen in people with hemiplegia during swing phase.

F. Frontal plane knee problems

Frontal Plane Knee Problems Table

1. **Excessive varus**—static factors: ligamentous laxity, weakness of lateral joint structures, trauma, and rickets; dynamic factors: malalignment due to osteoarthritis, tibial varum, and excessive foot supination.

2. **Excessive valgus**—static factors: laxity of medial ligaments, trauma, and weakness of medial joint structures; dynamic factors: hindfoot varus, paralytic gait, arthritis, and hip anteversion.

Answer Figure 3-6B-1.

Part 7. Clinical Gait Deviations

Section A

Answers to Figure 3-7A-1.

1. Inadequate flexion—seen during IC through LR, it is caused by weak quadriceps, a result of flat foot or forefoot contact, knee pain, quadriceps spasticity, or impaired proprioception. Significance: decreased shock absorption and decreased forward progression of the tibia; potentially damaging to posterior structures of the knee joint.

   Seen during PSw and ISw, it is caused by inadequate hip extension or absent heel off during TSt, knee pain, joint contracture, arthritis, a primitive extension pattern, extensor spasticity, or motor control problems. Significance: problems with thigh advancement starting in PSw and foot clearance during ISw, and difficulty in bringing the trailing limb closer to the body during early swing.

2. Excessive flexion—seen during IC through LR, it is caused by joint flexion contracture, hamstring or gastrocnemius spasticity, compensation for excessive ankle dorsiflexion or hip flexion, or impaired sensation. Significance: results in increased demand on quadriceps and destabilizes the knee. Excessive knee flexion during swing (ISw) is not functionally significant.

3. Inadequate extension—seen during MSt, it is caused by knee pain, joint contracture, secondary to inadequate hip extension, or excessive dorsiflexion or posterior pelvic tilt. Significance: puts increased demand on quadriceps and destabilizes the knee. Seen during terminal stance (TSt), the cause is usually to lower the body for a short opposite limb and this also puts increased demand on the quadriceps and destabilizes the knee. Seen during terminal swing (TSw), it is caused by joint contracture, hamstring or gastrocnemius contracture, hamstring spasticity, weak quadriceps, the result of the primitive flexion pattern, or motor control problems, or an attempt to decrease the demand on the hip extensors during LR or to accommodate forefoot or flat foot contact during IC. Significance: decreases step length of involved limb, hinders heel strike at IC.

4. Hyperextension—seen during IC through LR, it is caused by weak quadriceps, plantarflexion contractures or spasticity at the ankle, quadriceps spasticity, or intentional locking to stabilize the limb. Significance: decreases shock absorption, may interfere with heel rocker mechanism and forward progression of the tibia, may cause damage to posterior structures of the knee joint. Seen during midstance (MSt) and terminal stance (TSt), it is caused by excessive ankle plantarflexion, impaired proprioception, or an attempt to stabilize the limb. Significance: interferes with ankle rocker and forward progression of the tibia, may cause damage to posterior structures of the knee joint. Seen during swing, it is caused by a persistent extensor pattern, extensor spasticity, impaired proprioception, or voluntary activation of mass extension pattern to extend the knee. Significance: difficulty clearing the foot, and may cause damage to posterior structures of the knee joint.

5. Extensor thrust—seen during LR or early MSt, it is caused by extensor spasticity activating a total limb extension pattern, or voluntary activation of the quadriceps muscle to stabilize the knee. Significance: decreases shock absorption, may interfere with heel rocker mechanism and forward progression of the tibia, and may cause damage to posterior structures of the knee joint.

6. Wobble or buckling—seen during IC through LR, it is caused by impaired sensation. Significance: decreased forward momentum and decreased limb stability. Seen during MSt, it is caused by quadriceps weakness, plantarflexor weakness, and extensor spasticity. Significance: interferes with forward momentum, balance, and limb stability.

7. Excessive flexion as a contralateral compensation—seen during swing phase, it is caused by an attempt to clear the foot when the contralateral limb is too short functionally. Significance: puts increased demand on the hip and knee flexors of the swinging limb. Seen during single limb support, it is caused by an attempt to lower the body and enable a short contralateral limb to contact the ground. Significance: puts increased demand on the quadriceps and contributes to limb instability.

Part 8. Observational Gait Analysis—The Knee

Answers depend on individual lab groups.

Part 9. Thought Questions

1. With the foot fixed on the floor during stance phase, the limb functions as a closed kinematic chain. A contraction of the soleus muscle on a fixed foot will retract the tibia and extend the knee.

2. Women have wider hips than men. This puts a greater stress on the quadriceps muscle and increases the Q angle. This increased stress results in greater knee injuries in women athletes.

3. Forty-five degree flexion contractures at the knee will necessitate ankle dorsiflexion and hip flexion. The pelvic girdle may have an anterior tilt with an increased lumbar lordosis. Other possibilities are: a neutral pelvic girdle with forward trunk flexion or a posterior pelvic tilt and a dorsal kyphosis.

4. a. The resting position of a hot, swollen, painful knee is 30° of flexion.

   b. Anything to decrease the forces on this joint: shorter steps, decreased velocity, inadequate knee extension in TSw and TSt, inadequate knee flexion during PSw and ISw, lateral trunk lean over each stance limb, forward trunk lean, decreased heel rocker, decreased forefoot rocker, delayed heel rise until weight has shifted onto the contralateral limb, increased double limb support, and changes in arm swing.

   c. Increased pronation and medial weight-bearing.

   d. Footflat or low heel contact, hyperpronation throughout single limb support, decreased heel rise and delayed heel rise, and increased dorsiflexion during swing to clear toes.

   e. Increased hip flexion, adduction, and internal rotation. The pelvis may have an increased anterior tilt and the dorsal spine may have an increased lumbar lordosis. An alternative positioning may include a neutral pelvis with a forward trunk lean throughout the gait cycle and a lateral trunk lean toward each stance limb.

5. Plantarflexion at the ankle: decreased hip flexion, and a compensation at the pelvic girdle and dorsal spine to bring the GRFV as anterior as possible for balance.

6. Foot and ankle: lateral weight-bearing, feet supinated. Hip: abducted, externally rotated, and with decreased flexion. The pelvic girdle and dorsal spine may show a variety of compensations to maintain balance.

7. The knee may lock in extension or lock in flexion depending on where the loose body has lodged. The patient will report that the knee tends to give way during weight-bearing.

8. The knee may lock in extension or lock in flexion depending on where the tear is. The patient will report that the knee tends to lock or give way during weight-bearing.

Chapter 4
Normal and Pathological Hip Function
Part 1. Terminology

Section A

Motions of the Hip

1. Flexion—sagittal plane motion around an axis at the intersections of the frontal and transverse planes in which the distal aspects of both segments come closer together.

2. Extension—sagittal plane motion around an axis at the intersections of the frontal and transverse planes in which the distal aspects of both segments move farther apart.

3. Internal or medial rotation—transverse plane motion around an axis at the intersections of the sagittal and frontal planes in which the segments rotate toward the midline.

4. External or lateral rotation—transverse plane motion around an axis at the intersections of the sagittal and frontal planes in which the segments rotate away from the midline.

5. Adduction—frontal plane motion around an axis at the intersections of the sagittal and transverse planes in which the distal segment moves toward the body's midline.

6. Abduction—frontal plane motion around an axis at the intersections of the sagittal and transverse planes in which the distal segment moves away from the body's midline.

Section B

Deformities of the Hip

1. Coxa vara—frontal plane deformity in which there is a reduction in the angle between the neck and the shaft of the femur.

2. Coxa valga—frontal plane deformity in which there is an increase in the angle between the neck and the shaft of the femur.

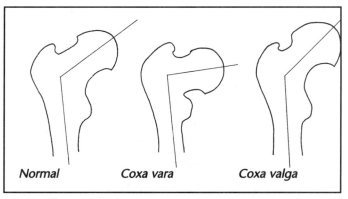

Answer Figure 4-1B-1.

3. Anteversion—transverse plane deformity in which the angle between the neck of the femur and the frontal plane is increased.

4. Retroversion—transverse plane deformity in which the angle between the neck of the femur and the frontal plane is decreased.

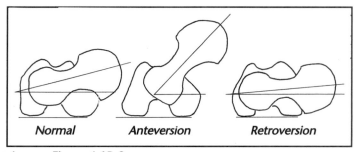

Answer Figure 4-1B-2.

5. Legg-Calvé-Perthes disease—osteochondrosis and osteonecrosis of the femoral epiphysial plate; occurs in children from 5 to 9 years of age, seen in boys more than girls. The patient may exhibit a psoas limp involving hip external rotation, adduction, and flexion with exaggerated pelvic and trunk movements to advance the thigh.

6. Slipped capital epiphysis—inferior and posterior subluxation or dislocation of femoral head; occurs in children aged 10 to 15, in twice as many boys as girls. The patient may exhibit an antalgic gait with affected externally rotated limb; pain may be referred to the knee.

7. Congenital hip dislocation—congenital subluxation or dislocation of the femoral head, usually the result of a shallow acetabulum.

Part 2. Normal Functional Anatomy

Section A

Osteology

1. Answers to Figure 4-2A-1:
   a. Greater trochanter
   b. Head
   c. Neck

d. Fovea

e. Lesser trochanter

f. Shaft

Answers to Figure 4-2A-2:

g. Ilium

h. Greater sciatic notch

i. Articular surface of acetabulum

j. Acetabular fossa

k. Pubis

l. Lesser sciatic notch

m. Obturator foramen

n. Ichium

2. a. Angle between the neck and the shaft of the femur.

b. Angle between the neck and the frontal plane.

c. Network of osseous tissue comprising the cancellous structure of a bone.

d. Area of decreased trabeculae in the femoral neck; in elderly, osteoporotic individuals the zone of weakness is a common site for femoral neck fractures.

Section B

Arthrology

1. Capsular pattern: the greatest limitation is in flexion and internal rotation, there is some limitation in abduction, there is no limitation in adduction or external rotation.

2. Maximal articular congruency: flexion, abduction, and lateral rotation.

3. Ligamentum teres serves as a conduit for blood and nerve supply to the femoral head.

4. Ball and socket joint with three degrees of freedom.

5. Anteriorly, the hip joint is supported by the iliofemoral ("Y" or Bigalow ligament) and pubofemoral ligaments.

6. Posteriorly, the hip joint is supported by the ischiofemoral ligament.

Part 3. Hip Movements and the Closed Kinematic Chain

Section A

Pelvic Girdle and Lumbar Spine Responses

<table>
<tr><td colspan="3" align="center">Response Table</td></tr>
<tr><td>Hip Movements</td><td>Pelvic Girdle Responses</td><td>Lumbar Spine Responses</td></tr>
<tr><td>1. Flexion</td><td>Anterior pelvic tilt</td><td>Increased lumbar extension</td></tr>
<tr><td>2. Extension</td><td>Posterior pelvic tilt</td><td>Lumbar flexion</td></tr>
<tr><td>3. Abduction</td><td>Contralateral pelvic hike</td><td>Contralateral lateral trunk flexion</td></tr>
<tr><td>4. Adduction</td><td>Contralateral pelvic drop</td><td>Ipsilateral lateral trunk flexion</td></tr>
<tr><td>5. Internal rotation</td><td>Contralateral pelvic forward rotation</td><td>Contralateral trunk rotation</td></tr>
<tr><td>6. External rotation</td><td>Contralateral pelvic backward rotation</td><td>Ipsilateral trunk rotation</td></tr>
</table>

Answer Figure 4-3A-1.

Section B

Knee, Ankle, and Foot Responses

<table>
<tr><td colspan="2" align="center">Response Table</td></tr>
<tr><td>Hip Movements</td><td>Knee, Ankle, Foot Responses</td></tr>
<tr><td>1. Flexion</td><td>Knee flexion, ankle dorsiflexion</td></tr>
<tr><td>2. Extension</td><td>Knee extension, ankle neutral to plantarflexion</td></tr>
<tr><td>3. Abduction</td><td>Abduction force at the knee, medial weight-bearing at the foot, wide base of support (BOS)</td></tr>
<tr><td>4. Adduction</td><td>May get adduction force at the knee, lateral weight-bearing at the foot, narrow BOS</td></tr>
<tr><td>5. Internal rotation</td><td>Stress on the lateral aspect of the knee, toe-in at the foot</td></tr>
<tr><td>6. External rotation</td><td>Stress on the medial aspect of the knee, increased toe-out at the foot</td></tr>
</table>

Answer Figure 4-3B-1.

Part 4. Normal Hip Function—Sagittal Plane

Section A

Kinematics

Curve describing the movement of the hip joint.

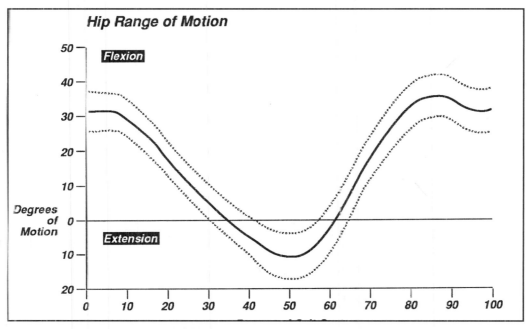

Answer Figure 4-4A-1. Reprinted from Perry.

Section B

Kinetics

Answers to Figure 4-4B-1: The muscles in consecutive order are: hip extensors: biceps femoris (long head), semimembranosis. semitendonosis, adductor magnus, gluteus maximus (lower fibers).

Answers to Figure 4-4B-2: hip adductors: adductor longus, adductor magnus, gracilis.

Answers to Figure 4-4B-3: hip abductors: gluteus medius, gluteus maximus (upper fibers), tensor fascia lata.

Answers to Figure 4-4B-4: hip flexors: adductor longus, rectus femoris, gracilis, sartorius, iliacus.

These results occur during the gait subdivisions.

5. Hip extensor muscles are working when the hip is flexed (initial contact [IC], loading response [LR] and midswing [MSw] through terminal swing [TSw]). Hip flexors are working during preswing (PSw) and initial swing (ISw) to clear the foot.

Gait Subdivision Table	
1. Maximal hip flexion (ROM)	Between ISw and MSw
2. Maximal hip extension (ROM)	TSt
3. Extensor muscle activity (MMT)	IC, LR, MSw, TSw
4. Flexor muscle activity (MMT)	TSt, PSw, ISw

Answer Figure 4-4B-5. ROM = range of motion; ISw = initial swing; MSw = midswing; TSt = terminal stance; MMT = manual muscle test; IC = intial contact; LR = loading response; TSw = terminal swing; PSw = preswing; ISw = initial swing.

Part 5. Normal Hip Function—Frontal Plane

Section A

1. Maximal hip abduction occurs at ISw. The pelvis drops as the swing limb comes off the ground resulting in a relative abduction of the hip with respect to the pelvis.

2. Maximal hip adduction occurs at IC. As the training limb unweights the foot, the pelvis dips to the side of the trailing limb. This results in a relative adduction of the hip on the side experiencing IC.

3. Curve describing hip joint movement in the frontal plane.

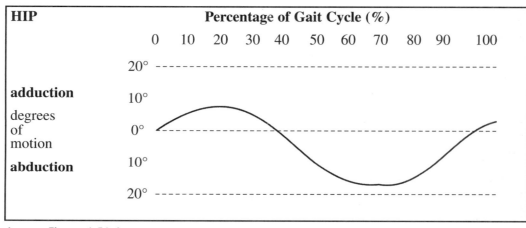

Answer Figure 4-5A-1.

Part 6. Normal Hip Function—Transverse Plane

At IC the thigh is neutral. Maximal internal rotation occurs during LR and then the limb starts to externally rotate. Maximal external rotation occurs at PSw and then the hip internally rotates during swing. The full arc of movement is approximately 8°.

Some factors that cause transverse plane hip motion include hindfoot pronation and supination, internal and external rotation at the knee and forward and backward rotation of the pelvic girdle.

Part 7. Hip Pathomechanics

Graph of abnormal hip function.

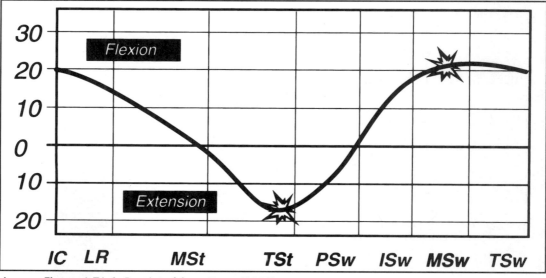

Answer Figure 4-7A-1. Reprinted from Perry (1992).

Section A

Inadequate Extension

1. Midstance (MSt) through ISw.

2. Demonstrate the gait deviations.

3. Arthrodesis with hip fixed in 20° to 40° of flexion, joint contracture, iliotibial band contracture, hip flexor spasticity, pain (hip flexes to approximately 30° to minimize intra-articular pressure), as a compensation for knee flexion or hyperextension, as a compensation for excessive ankle plantarflexion, and fixed anterior pelvic tilt.

Section 3

Excessive Flexion

1. Demonstrate the gait deviations.

2. Weak hip flexor muscles, arthrodesis, joint contracture, iliotibial band contracture, hip flexor spasticity, pain (hip flexes to approximately 30° to minimize intra-articular pressure), as a compensation for knee flexion or hyperextension, as a compensation for excessive ankle plantarflexion, and fixed anterior pelvic tilt.

Section C

Inadequate Flexion

1. IC, LR, ISw, MSw.

2. End of terminal stance (TSt), PSw, ISw, and the beginning of MSw.

3. Demonstrate and describe the gait deviations.

Section D

Other Hip Deviations in the Sagittal Plane

1. Many hip compensations are possible to help with foot clearance: increased hip flexion during swing, hip hiking, and hip circumduction.

2. With weak quadriceps, hip compensations help to stabilize the knee at IC and MSt including: increasing hip flexion to put the ground reaction force vector anterior to the knee, creating an extension moment, or externally rotating the limb during stance to decrease the knee's ability to flex during gait.

3. A fixed anterior pelvic tilt will cause excessive hip flexion and inadequate hip extension.

4. A fixed posterior pelvic tilt will cause decreased hip flexion.

Section E

Hip Problems in the Frontal and Transverse Planes

1. Coxa vara means that the angle of inclination is lower than the normal 120° to 130° adult value. A fixed coxa vara would cause a relative shortening of the limb with thigh adduction, an abduction (valgus) force at the knee and medial weight-bearing, and pronation at the foot. If the femur has a coxa vara deformity but the joint is free to move, tightness in the hip abductor muscles may result in hip abduction, an adduction (varus) force at the knee and supination with lateral weight-bearing at the foot.

2. Coxa valga means that the angle of inclination is greater than the normal 120° to 130° adult value. This condition causes a relative lengthening of the affected limb and shortens the lever arm for the hip abductors. If the head of the femur is fixed in the acetabulum, the thigh would be abducted creating an abduction (varus) force at the knee with supination and lateral weight-bearing at the foot. If the head of the femur can move, the shortened lever arm for the hip abductors may cause a gluteus medius limp and an abduction (valgus) moment at the knee with medial weight-bearing, and pronation at the foot.

3. Hip anteversion means that the angle of femoral torsion is increased. On the affected limb, this condition may cause a medially deviated patella (*squinting patella*) or a reduced or absent toe-out. Patients report knee pain and a history of lateral patellar subluxations.

Section F

Clinical Problems

1. Hip abductor weakness—the pelvic girdle will fall to the contralateral side during IC, LR, and single limb support.

2. Hip adductor contracture—the hip cannot abduct during ISw. The width of base of support (BOS) may narrow or the patient may laterally trunk lean away from the affected limb during swing to compensate for the lack of adduction.

3. Hip adductor spasticity—depending on the severity of the spasticity, the hip may be held in flexion, adduction, and internal rotation. To advance the affected limb, the patient may rotate the pelvic girdle backward on the affected side enabling the hip adductors to substitute for hip flexors (see Walker 1 on the companion videotape).

4. Iliotibial band tightness—can cause excessive hip flexion and inadequate extension at the hip with the thigh adducted or increased abduction (valgus) at the knee.

5. Knee flexion contracture—can cause excessive hip flexion and inadequate extension at the hip.

6. Pain due to arthritis in the joint will limit joint motion and reflexly inhibit muscle action. The hip's position of least intra-articular pressure is 30° flexion.

7. A cane in the contralateral hand has a relatively long moment arm so even with 10% of the patient's body weight going through the cane the reduction of forces at the painful hip can be considerable.

Part 8. Gait Deviations

Section A

Answers to Figure 4-8A-1.

1. Inadequate flexion—seen during IC and LR, it is caused by an attempt to reduce the demand on the hip extensors, problems in TSw with limited hip flexion or the past retract mechanism. Significance: may interfere with LR by limiting knee flexion and ankle plantarflexion. Seen during swing, it is caused by weak hip flexors, hip pain, joint contracture, tight hamstring muscles, hip extensor spasticity, and a prolonged primitive extensor pattern. Significance: difficulty with foot clearance, limb advancement, forward momentum, and shortened step length.

2. Excessive flexion—seen during IC and LR, it is caused by hip flexion contracture, weak hip extensors, flexor spasticity, iliotibial band contracture, arthrodesis, pain, and a compensation for excessive ankle dorsiflexion with increased knee flexion. Significance: increased demand on quadriceps with knee flexed, decreases limb stability. Seen during swing, there is compensation to aid with foot clearance if the swinging limb is functionally too long (may be due to actual leg length discrepancy, plantarflexion contracture, or inadequate knee flexion). Significance: increased energy cost but helps with foot clearance.

3. Inadequate extension—seen during late MSt and TSt, it is caused by hip flexion contracture, arthrodesis, pain, iliotibial band contracture, excessive knee flexion with ankle dorsiflexion, and compensation for a plantarflexion contracture. Significance: places increased demand on quadriceps and hip extensors, decreases step length of contralateral limb, decreases limb stability.

4. Past thigh retraction—seen during swing, a maneuver that involves a quick hip flexion followed by a rapid thigh retraction to snap the knee into extension and lock the joint in its close-packed position in preparation for weight-bearing at IC. Significance: two groups of patients use this maneuver—people with weak, flaccid, or unstable knees (i.e., people with polio, people insecure on prosthetic knees) and people with spasticity and primitive flexion and extension patterns.

5. Excessive internal rotation—seen throughout the gait cycle, it is caused by femoral anteversion, adductor spasticity, contracture or spasticity of the internal rotators, and joint contracture. Significance: may cause lateral stress on the knee if it occurs during weight-bearing, in-toeing, or difficulty with forward progression and foot clearance during swing.

6. Excessive external rotation—seen during weight-bearing, it is caused by a joint contracture, a muscle contracture, an attempt to stabilize a weak knee, or an attempt to reduce forces on a painful forefoot. Significance: increases width of BOS, causes an increase in toe-out, decreases forefoot rocker, may stress the medial aspect of the knee joint. Seen during swing, it is caused by attempts to advance the limb by substituting hip adductors for weak hip flexors or attempts to functionally shorten the limb or forefoot. Significance: may assist with foot clearance and limb advancement.

7. Excessive abduction—seen during single limb support, it is caused by a functionally longer reference limb, abduction contracture, and obesity. Significance: it functionally shortens the limb, and widens the BOS. Seen during swing, it is caused by abduction contracture, efforts to clear the long limb, and obesity. Significance: assists foot clearance.

8. Excessive adduction—seen throughout the gait cycle, it is caused by adductor spasticity, adductor contractures, and Legg-Calvé-Perthes disease. Significance: it decreases limb stability and BOS, makes the limb functionally longer, and may interfere with foot clearance during swing.

Part 9. Observational Gait Analysis—The Hip
Answers depend on individual lab groups.

Part 10. Thought Questions
Section A

1. The lowest level in which complete innervation exists.

2. The left extremity muscles that are still functioning in a patient with an L_3 lesion:

Trunk: quadratus lumborum T_{12} to L_1, rectus abdominus—intercostal nerves T_{7-12}, external and internal obliques T_8 to T_{12}, L_1

Hip:
Flexors: psoas major $L_{2,3}$, iliacus $L_{2,3}$

Flexors with rotation: sartorius $L_{2,3}$

Extensors: none

Abductors: none

Adductors: pectineus $L_{2,3,4}$, addus magnus $L_{3,4}$, addus brevis $L_{3,4}$, addus longus $L_{3,4}$, gracilis $L_{3,4}$

External rotation: obturator externus $L_{3,4}$ only

Internal rotators: None

Knee:
Flexion: none

Extension: quadriceps femoris (rectus femoris and vasti) L_{2-4}

Ankle and foot: none

3. Hip, knee, and ankle joint problems.

Joint	Problem	Explanation
Hip	Hip flexion and adduction contractures	Muscles are unopposed; patient spends lots of time sitting with hips flexed
Knee	Genu recurvatum Lock knee in extension on weight bearing Knee flexion contractures	Weak quadriceps; no hamstrings
Ankle/foot	Plantarflexion contractures	Patient sitting in wheel chair; tight gastrocnemius tight heelcords; increased time in bed

Answer Figure 4-10A-1.

159

4. The patient is also at risk for developing decubiti, deconditioning, muscle atrophy, osteoporosis, and hip flexion and adduction-contractures. If the patient did not have any joint contractures, he or she could walk with bilateral solid ankle foot orthosis. The patient has good potential to be a household ambulator but may need a wheelchair for community mobility. The physical therapy program should include strengthening of the remaining musculatures, functional activities, and orthotics training. Creative gait training programs are to be encouraged.

Chapter 5
Normal and Pathological Kinematics and Kinetics—Head, Arms, and Torso
Part 1. Normal Head, Arms, and Trunk Function
Section A
Displacement of the Center of Gravity

1. a. Single limb support (mid-stance [MSt]).

   b. Double limb support.

   c. Two to four inches.

   d. Strategies for minimizing the center of gravity (COG) vertical displacement—contralateral pelvic drop, horizontal pelvic forward rotation, lateral pelvic displacement, ankle placement during double limb support, interaction between ankle and knee motion, and substitution of inertia for complete frontal plane alignment of the COG over the base of support (BOS).

2. a. Right MSt.

   b. Left MSt.

   c. Two inches; approximately one inch to each side.

   d. Lateral pelvic shift toward the stance limb, horizontal pelvic forward rotation, substitution of inertia for complete frontal plane alignment of the COG over the BOS.

Section B
Pelvic Girdle Movement

1. Recall the pelvic movements in three planes during gait:

   a. Sagittal: anterior and posterior

   b. Frontal: pelvic dip and hike (or pelvic drop and rise)

   c. Transverse: forward and backward rotation

2. What is the normal range of motion (ROM) for pelvic motion in each plane during gait?

   a. Sagittal: 7°

   b. Frontal: 4°

   c. Transverse: 10° (Hoppenfeld says 40°)

   d. Answers refer to individual lab groups.

3. Write down and test your hypothesis.

Part 2. Shoulder Girdle and Upper Extremity Function

1. Shoulders provide counter rotation for the pelvis to improve balance by arranging the body parts around the body's COG.

2. Arm ROM

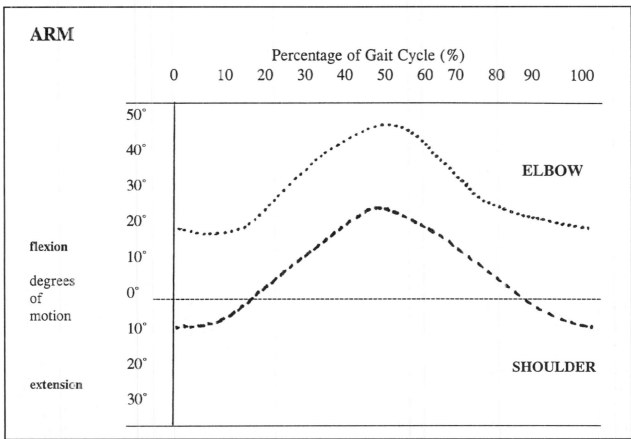

Answer Figure 5-2A-1. Adapted from Murray, M. P., Sepic, S. B., & Bernard, E. J. (1967). Patterns of sagittal rotation of the upper limbs in walking. Physical Therapy, 47, 272-284. Reprinted from Perry (1992).

3. In order the muscles are: upper trapezius, supraspinatus, posterior deltoid, middle deltoid, and teres major.

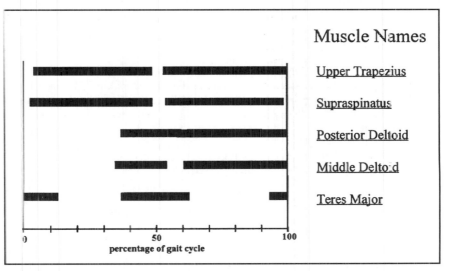

Answer Figure 5-2A-2.

Part 3. Head, Arms, and Torso and Variations in Gait Parameters

Section A

Answers refer to individual lab groups.

Section B

Analysis

Based on your observations in the previous sections make some generalizations about the role of gait in the following:

1. Arm—used for balance and forward momentum.

2. Head—used for righting and equilibrium.

3. Trunk—balance and momentum.

4. Pelvic girdle—increased rotation to change width of BOS.

Part 4. Pathological Gaits

Section A

Answers to Figure 5-4A-1.

1. Backward trunk lean—seen during stance phase, it is caused by an attempt to decrease the demand on the hip extensors. Significance: may increase energy cost and decrease forward momentum. Seen during swing phase, it is caused by an attempt to advance the limb. Significance: may increase energy cost.

2. Forward trunk lean—seen during stance, it is caused by abdominal pain, a postural problem with the dorsal spine (i.e., kyphosis, ankylosing spondylitis), a hip problem involving excessive flexion (seen during initial contact [IC] and loading response [LR]), or inadequate hip extension (seen during late midstance [MSt] and terminal stance [TSt]), a compensation for weak hip extensors (slight forward trunk flexion puts hip extensors in more optimal range), an attempt to bring the ground reaction force vector anterior to stabilize weak knee extensors, an attempt to maintain forward progression over an excessively plantarflexed ankle, or an attempt to substitute visual placing for decreased proprioception. Significance: increases energy cost and may increase demand on hip extensors.

3. Lateral trunk lean—seen during IC and LR, it is caused by weak hip abductors. Significance: may increase energy cost and decrease forward momentum. Seen during single limb support, it is caused by an attempt to decrease forces on a painful hip. Significance: may increase energy cost and decrease forward momentum. Seen during swing phase, it is caused by leg length discrepancy, an attempt to clear a swinging limb, and synergy with a cane. Significance: may increase energy cost and decrease forward momentum.

4. Trunk with backward rotation—seen during stance phase, it is caused by motor control problems in which trunk movements cannot be disassociated from the pelvic or extremity movements, a strategy used by people with motor control problems to position the limb so hip adductors can be substituted for hip flexors to advance the affected limb. Significance: may increase energy cost, decrease stability, and decrease forward momentum. Seen during swing phase, it is caused by synergy with a cane, compensation to clear the foot if the ankle had excessive plantarflexion during single limb support. Significance: may increase energy cost, decrease stability, and decrease forward momentum.

5. Trunk with forward rotation—seen during stance phase, it is caused by motor control problems in which trunk movements cannot be disassociated from the pelvic or extremity movements. Significance: may increase energy cost and decrease stability. Seen during swing phase, it is caused by synergy with a cane or strategy to advance the limb. Significance: may increase energy cost and decrease stability.

6. Increased lumbar lordosis—seen during stance phase, it is caused by flexion contracture of the hip joint, hip flexor spasticity, weakness of abdominal or hip extensor muscles, and an increased anterior pelvic tilt. Significance: may increase energy cost and decrease stability.

7. Hip hiking—seen during swing, it is caused by an attempt to clear the swinging limb. Significance: may increase energy cost.

8. Posterior pelvic tilt—seen throughout the gait cycle, it is caused by low back pain, tight hamstrings, limited lumbar extension, an attempt to decrease demand on the hip extensors (IC and LR), and a strategy to advance the limb (initial swing [ISw] and midswing [MSw]). Significance: may increase energy cost, may cause knee flexion during MSt and TSt, and destabilize the limb.

9. Anterior pelvic tilt—seen throughout the gait cycle, it is caused by flexion contracture of the hip joint, hip flexor spasticity, weakness of the abdominal or hip extensor muscles, and may be associated with an anterior trunk lean or an increased lumbar lordosis. Significance: may increase energy cost and result in low back pain.

10. Reduced or absent forward pelvic rotation—seen during IC and LR, it is caused by back pain, motor control problems in which trunk movements cannot be disassociated from the pelvic or extremity movements, an attempt to decrease demand on the quadriceps and hip extensors, and a lack of contralateral pelvic rotation. Significance: decreases step length. Seen during swing, it is caused by back pain, motor control problems, and a lack of contralateral pelvic rotation. Significance: decreases step length.

11. Reduced or absent backward pelvic rotation—seen throughout the gait cycle, it is caused by motor control problems of the trunk and pelvis and back pain. Significance: decreases the contralateral step length.

12. Excessive backward pelvic rotation—seen throughout the gait cycle, it is caused by a strategy to advance the limb, motor control problems in which pelvic movements cannot be disassociated from extremity movements, and compensation for excessive ankle plantarflexion. Significance: may decrease limb advancement and interfere with forward progression.

13. Ipsilateral pelvic drop—seen during stance, it is caused by a short reference limb. Significance: may cause back pain. Seen during swing, it is caused by weak contralateral hip abductors, voluntary to lower limb for IC. Significance: may increase energy cost, may destabilize the contralateral limb, and enables relative lengthening of the reference limb.

14. Contralateral pelvic drop—seen during IC and LR, it is caused by weak hip abductors of the reference limb and is voluntary to the lower limb for IC. Significance: may increase energy cost, may destabilize the reference limb, and enables relative lengthening of the contralateral limb. Seen during swing, it is caused by a short reference limb. Significance: may cause back pain.

Part 5. Observational Gait Analysis—The Head, Arms, and Torso

Answers refer to individual lab groups.

Part 6. Thought Questions

1. a. Hips: increased flexion; lumbar spine: increased lordosis.

   b. Gait deviations seen throughout gait cycle may include: excessive hip flexion, inadequate hip extension, an anterior trunk lean or an increased lumbar lordosis, decreased knee flexion or increased knee extension, increased ankle plantarflexion and a decrease in ankle dorsiflexion, and maybe an increase in energy cost and complaints of back pain.

2. a. Right pelvis high.

   b. Gait deviations are a functional leg length discrepancy with the right leg short and the left leg long. During swing, the body must develop a strategy to clear the left leg. Possibilities include: lateral trunk lean to the right, abduction of the left limb, circumduction of left limb, increased left hip and knee flexion, and increased left ankle dorsiflexion with increased toe dorsiflexion. During stance on the right side, the functionally shorter limb can compensate by increasing plantarflexion, decreasing hip and knee flexion, and decreasing the step length or vaulting.

3. T_{12} spinal cord lesion.

   a. Functional muscles: rectus abdominus, rectus obliquis, may have partial innervation of internal oblique, external oblique, transverse abdominis, may have partial innervation of erector spinae, may have partial innervation of quadratus lumborum, no lower extremity muscles but can substitute latissimus dorsi for quadratus lumborum by using an assistive device and reverse action of the muscle.

   b. Many programs are possible. Include training for static and dynamic balance, transfers, a gait progression from parallel bars to assistive devices, and an orthotics management program. The patient could benefit from a knee-ankle-foot orthosis (such as a Scott-Craig orthosis) with solid ankles and knee locks.

   c. Abdominal muscles and latissimus dorsi can be used for limb advancement.

   d. The patient can use a swing-to, a swing-through, or a 2-point or a 4-point gait pattern.

   e. Independent ambulation for household use is reasonable. A wheelchair would be recommended for community mobility. Factors to consider include: age, strength, endurance, athleticism, motivation, cardiovascular fitness, medical condition, sensation, joint mobility and contractures, premorbid condition, amount of spasticity, attention and cognitive factors, and safety issues.

Chapter 6
Gait Through the Life Span
Part 1. Terminology

1. High guard—upper extremity positioning seen during the gait of children who have just begun walking independently. The thoracic spine is extended; the scapulae are adducted; the shoulders are elevated, flexed, and abducted; and often the elbows are flexed and the hands are either fisted or carrying objects.

2. Primitive patterns—a term used to describe the flexion and extension synergies seen in the extremities of people with neurological deficits. The word "primitive" is used because total limb flexion and extension synergies are seen during the first year of normal development.

3. Pattern generator—the theoretical part of the central nervous system that formulates the movement of muscles which are functionally linked together (in patterns). This idea hypothesizes a mechanism for decreasing the complexity of motor activity.

4. Astasia—the period of time during normal development (usually between 2-4 months) when a child will not bear weight if held in a standing position.

5. Abasia—the period of time during normal development (usually between 2-4 months) when a child will not bear weight or demonstrate stepping if held upright in a walking position.

6. Reflex—a stereotypical response to a given and adequate stimulus.

7. Equilibrium reaction—according to the reflex-hierarchy theories, these are balance reactions that enable the body to control the center of gravity (COG) through space. Three types of equilibrium reactions are described: postural fixations, which enable the body to hold a given position; tilting reactions, which permit the body to maintain its balance even when the base of support (BOS) is moving; and protective extension reactions, which facilitate extension tone in the appropriate extremities to catch the body when it is falling and guard it from injury.

8. Associated movements—the activation of muscle groups during increased effort that are not directly related to the functional task (i.e., during the lifting of a very heavy object, the platysma muscle may get activated).

9. Cruising—a precursor to independent ambulation. A child walks holding onto furniture for stability.

10. Muscle tone—a "force with which a muscle resists being lengthened...its stiffness" (Shumway-Cook & Woollacott, 1995, p. 125).

11. Dynamical system—a system of the body that is complex, cooperative, self-organizing, and develops in an asynchronous and nonlinear manner. As a result of the asynchrony and nonlinear development of each system, motor milestones appear to emerge abruptly when all of the systems are sufficiently mature for the task.

12. Integration—according to the reflex-hierarchy theories, the time when the developmental reflex can no longer be elicited using the stimulus, and the pattern of movement associated with the reflex is now part of the individual's nervous system and available for voluntary use. Under stressful circumstances, even reflexes that have integrated can re-emerge.

13. Feedback—a system in which the body gets sensory input about how well it has accomplished a motor task and can modify its responses to improve the motor output on the next trial.

14. Feed forward—a system in which we anticipate a motor task and mentally rehearse it before actually attempting it.

15. Ankle and hip strategies—movement patterns that restore a person's COG to a stable position after perturbation. Small perturbations result in activation of the ankle muscles. Large perturbations result in activation of the hip musculature.

Part 2. Motor Control Foundations for Mature Gait

Section A

Developmental Reflexes

The following section has been adapted with permission from these three sources: Barnes, M. R., Crutchfield, C. A., & Heriza, C. B. (1977). The neurophysiological basis of patient treatment (Vol. II). *Reflexes in motor development*. Morgantown, WV: Stokesville Publishing Co.

Vulpe, S. G. (1977). *Vulpe assessment battery* (pp. 345-355). Toronto, Ontario: The National Institute on Mental Retardation. Updated edition available from Solsson Educational Publications, POB 280, E Aurora, New York, NY 14052.

Fiorentino, M. R. (1973). *Reflex testing methods for evaluating C.N.S. development* (2nd ed.). Springfield, Ill: Charles C. Thomas, Publisher, Ltd.

Answers to Figure 6-2A-1.

1. Flexor withdrawal
   Onset: begins at 28 weeks gestation.
   Integration: 2 months.
   Description: place the child supine with the head in the midline and the legs relaxed. Administer a noxious stimulus, such as a pin prick, to the sole of one foot and look for mass flexion of the stimulated leg to escape from the provocation.
   Significance for gait: a possible reflex basis for the primitive flexion pattern seen during swing phase in people with neurological lesions.

2. Crossed extension
   Onset: begins at 28 weeks gestation.
   Integration 1 to 2 months.
   Description: place the child supine with the head in the midline and the lower extremities extended, hold one knee in extension while applying firm pressure to sole of the ipsilateral foot. The contralateral lower extremity flexion should adduct and extend as if to push the examiner's hand away.
   Significance for gait: a possible reflex basis for reciprocal activation of the lower extremities.

3. Plantar grasp
   Onset: begins at 28 weeks gestation.
   Integration: 9 months.
   Description: place the child supine with the head in the midline with the legs relaxed. Apply firm pressure against the plantar surface of the infant's foot, over the metatarsal heads. A positive response is plantarflexion of all the toes.
   Significance for gait: when this reflex integrates the child is ready for independent ambulation.

4. Neonatal positive supporting reaction left extremity (LE)
   Onset: begins at 35 weeks gestation.
   Integration: 1 to 2 months.
   Description: support the infant in the vertical position holding him or her under the arms and around the chest, let both feet make firm contact with a flat surface. The child should simultaneously contract the lower extremity flexor and extensor muscles, enabling weight-bearing with only a minimal amount of body weight. The neonatal version of a positive supporting reaction is partial flexion of the hips and knees.
   Significance for gait: considered to be a prerequisite for spontaneous stepping reflex; a possible reflex basis for the primitive extension pattern. When integration occurs the period of *astasia* (negative support) begins.

5. Spontaneous stepping
   Onset: begins at 27 weeks gestation.
   Integration: 2 months.
   Description: support the infant in the vertical position holding him or her securely under the arms and around the chest. Let the child's feet touch the table surface and incline the child forward. The child will make alternating, rhythmical and coordinated stepping movements. Gently move the child forward to accompany any stepping.
   Significance for gait: reciprocal mass flexion and extension patterns in a weight-bearing situation.

6. Proprioceptive placing LE
   Onset: begins at 35 weeks of gestation.
   Integration: 2 months.
   Description: hold the child in a vertical position supporting him or her under the arms and around the chest. Press the dorsum of one foot against the edge of a table. The infant's limb should flex at the knee and hip to lift the foot above the table. The leg should then extend and place the foot on the table top.
   Significance for gait: we need proprioceptive foot placement for mature gait.

7. Asymmetric tonic neck reflex (ATNR)
   Onset: birth to 2 months.
   Integration: 4 to 6 months.
   Description: place the child supine with the head in the midline, turn his or her head to one side and wait a moment. Flexion posturing should occur in the upper extremity on the skull side and extension posturing should occur in the upper extremity on the face side. Lower extremities can show a similar posturing.
   Significance for gait: if this reflex persists or is obligatory, it will interfere with balance and impede the acquisition of normal gait.

165

8. Tonic labyrinthine reflex (TLR) prone and supine
   Onset: birth and integration at 6 months.
   Description: position the child prone and then supine and observe the response. A positive finding is: in prone, flexor tone dominates and the child will not be able to lift his or her head or support weight on the arms; in supine, extensor tone dominates and the child will not be able to flex in a pull-to-sit test.
   Significance for gait: a persistence of this reflex will interfere with coordinated activation of flexor and extensor muscles.

9. Symmetrical tonic neck reflex (STNR)
   Onset: 4 to 6 months.
   Integration: 10 to 12 months.
   Description: place the child prone over your lap or put the child in a four-point position. Gently and passively flex and extend the child's head. Forward head flexion should produce flexion of the upper extremities and extension of the lower extremities. Extension of the head should produce extension of the upper extremities and flexion of the lower extremities.
   Significance for gait: persistence of this reflex will interfere with a reciprocal gait pattern and selective motor control of specific muscle groups.

Righting Reactions

10. Labyrinthine head righting
    Onset: birth to 2 months.
    No integration: persists throughout life.
    Description: blindfold the child and hold him or her vertically under the chest and arms. Now tilt the body gently anteriorly, posteriorly, and to both sides. The child's head should remain upright and oriented so the eyes are parallel to the horizon.
    Significance for gait: a person needs to maintain an upright posture to move through space.

11. Optical righting
    Onset: birth to 2 months is complete by 8 months.
    Integration: persists throughout life.
    Description: hold the child vertically under the chest and both arms. Now tilt the body anteriorly, posteriorly, and to both sides. The child's head should remain upright and oriented so the eyes are parallel to the horizon.
    Significance for gait: a person needs to maintain an upright posture to move through space.

12. Body righting reaction acting on the head (BOH)
    Onset: birth to 2 months, completely established by 8 months.
    Integration: persists throughout life.
    Description: this is the proprioceptive version of the righting reaction and is difficult to isolate from the labyrinthine and optical versions.
    Significance for gait: the body uses the redundant information gathered from the labyrinthine, optical, and tactile systems to help it maintain an upright posture.

13. Mature neck on body righting (NOB)
    Onset: 4 to 6 months.
    Integration: 5 years old when the child can get to standing without rotation.
    Description: place the child supine with the head in the midline. Now gently flex the child's head and turn it to one side until the chin is over the shoulder. The child's body should segmentally turn in the direction of the head until the child is side-lying. Repeat on the opposite side to see if you get a symmetrical response.
    Significance for gait: it indicates that the child has developed rotation around body axis which is necessary for coordinated trunk and pelvic movements during mature gait. Reflex must integrate for the coordinated movements to occur.

14. Mature body on body righting (BOB)
    Onset: 4 to 6 months.
    Integration: at 5 years old when the child can get to standing without rotation.
    Description: place the child supine with the head in the midline, flex one leg over the torso and rotate it across the pelvis to the opposite side. The child should roll segmentally with the pelvic girdle first, followed by the trunk, the shoulder girdle, and then the head toward the side of the flexed leg.
    Significance for gait: it indicates that the child has developed rotation around the body axis which is necessary for coordinated trunk and pelvic movements during mature gait. Reflex must integrate for the coordinated movements to occur.

Equilibrium Reactions

15. Visual placing LE
    Onset: 3 to 5 months.
    Integration: persists throughout life.
    Description: hold the child vertically with your hands under the arms and around the chest. Lower the child toward a supporting surface. The child should look at the surface and place one or both feet on top of it.
    Significance for gait: people use visual placing of their lower extremities if their proprioceptive system is impaired.

16. Parachute reaction
    Onset: 4 months.
    Integration: persists throughout life.
    Description: hold the child vertically around the waist and then lower the child rapidly toward a supporting surface feet first. Both legs should externally rotate and abduct, and the feet should dorsiflex in preparation for standing.
    Significance for gait: a necessary protective response for breaking falls, and a necessary reaction in preparation for independent standing.

17. a. Protective extension forward upper extremity (UE)
    Onset: 5 to 7 months.
    Integration: persists throughout life.
    Description: hold the child vertically around the waist then lower the child rapidly toward a supporting surface head first. The child should extend and abduct his or her arms with fingers spread open ready to break the fall.
    Significance for gait: necessary for catching oneself if falling to prevent injury.

    b. Protective extension sideways UE
    Onset: 7 months.
    Integration: persists throughout life.
    Description: have the child sit comfortably. Push the child rapidly to one side so as to displace the child's COG. The child will lose his or her balance. The arm closest to the ground should abduct and extend at the elbow, wrist, and hand in preparation for bearing weight and breaking the fall. Weight is taken on the open palm and fingers.
    Significance for gait: necessary for catching oneself if falling to prevent injury.

    c. Protective extension backwards UE
    Onset: 9 to 10 months.
    Integration: persists throughout life.
    Description: have the child sit comfortably. Push the child rapidly backward with enough force to displace the COG and off-set balance. In response, the child should extend both arms backward. The palms should open in preparation of bearing weight and breaking the fall.
    Significance for gait: necessary for balance and trunk rotation.

18. Postural fixation in standing
    Onset: 12 to 21 months.
    Integration: persists throughout life.
    Description: have the child stand and remain standing. You will push the child gently but firmly in all directions in an effort to displace the child's COG. The child should be able to maintain this posture without losing balance.
    Significance for gait: this reflex is important for maintaining one's COG and balance during standing and walking.

19. Tilting reaction in standing
    Onset: 12 to 21 months.
    Integration: persists throughout life.
    Description: have the child stand on an equilibrium (rocker) board. The child should be able to rock the board while standing on it and not fall over. As the child tilts from side to side, the spine should laterally flex toward the high side of the board. The lower leg should extend and the upper leg should flex. The process should reverse as the board tilts to the opposite side. The arms may abduct and extend. As the child tilts forward, the spine should extend with leg extension and ankle plantarflexion. The arms may abduct and extend. In response to a posterior tilt, the child's spine should flex with leg flexion and ankle dorsiflexion. Arms are flexed at the shoulders and extended at the elbows.
    Significance for gait: necessary for controlling one's COG through space, especially when walking over uneven or unstable surfaces.

20. Protective staggering LE

Onset: 15 to 18 months.

Integration: persists throughout life.

Description: have the child stand on a good supporting surface. Gently displace the child's COG in all directions. The child should sidestep, cross one foot in front of the other or do whatever correction is required to restore the displaced COG.

Significance for gait: enables control of COG in all directions if suddenly disrupted, very important for safe, independent ambulation.

Section B

Pattern Generator Theories

1. Similarities include the hierarchical command structure, the presence of specific movement patterns, and the fact that the "hold" and the "move" programs are very similar to the equilibrium reactions. Differences center around the fact that reflexes need a stimulus to get the response but pattern generators allow for spontaneous movement.

2. Nashner and his colleagues (Nashner, 1977; Nashner & Woollacott, 1979; and Hovak & Nashner, 1986) described movement patterns called "strategies" that help people maintain their upright position during perturbed stance. An ankle strategy is used when perturbation of balance is small. A hip strategy is used when the perturbations are large. Forward sway occurs after a backward perturbation. The gastrocnemius, hamstring, and lumbar paraspinal muscles are activated. A forward perturbation results in a backward sway with activation of the tibialis anterior, quadriceps, and abdominal muscles.

3. Sensory input is not necessary for movement.

4. Many answers are possible.

5. The neurological lesion could be causing program errors. There are two kinds of program errors: errors in selecting the right program or errors in executing the program correctly. People with neurological lesions could demonstrate one or both of these kinds of errors.

Section C

Servomechanism Theory

1. A closed-loop model requires feedback and error correction. Any answer that includes these elements is acceptable.

2. An open-loop model uses feed forward to plan and modify the movement before it occurs.
   Any answer including these elements is acceptable.

Section D

Dynamical System Theory

1. Basic concepts—answers refer to individual lab groups.

2. a. Flexion withdrawal.

    b. Asymmetric tonic neck reflex.

    c. Tilting reaction in standing.

    d. Protective staggering if you move, postural fixation in standing if you hold your ground.

3. Review the appropriate sections in the preceding chapters for answers to questions a-j.
   k. The developing child has a variety of joint constraints that limit movement. During the neonatal period the infant exhibits physiological flexion restricting joint motion. A tight joint synchrony is seen between the ankle, knee, and hip joints of the newborn but decreases over the first year of life, permitting more selective joint movement.

4. Postural control

    a. Answers refer to individual lab groups.

    b. Answers refer to individual lab groups.

    c. Wide BOS, slow velocity, rhythmic disturbances to cadence, uneven and inconsistent step lengths.

    d. Times vary from child to child. These are general guidelines—prone: 6 months; supine: 7 to 8 months; sitting: 7 to 8 months; standing: 12 to 15 months.

e. Dynamic and static equilibrium is essential for movement through space. Control of one's COG is a necessary component for mature gait.

5. Body constraints

a. When compared with adults, children have relatively larger heads, shorter limb lengths, higher mean angles of the femoral neck and shaft, increased femoral torsion, increased tibial torsion, and decreased ratios of pelvic width to leg length (this means that they have a proportionately wider BOS than adults).

b. Body constraints in the child reduce the step length, stride length, and velocity. The decreased ratios of pelvic width to leg length result in a proportionately wider BOS than adults. The higher mean angles of the femoral neck and shaft, increased femoral torsion, and increased tibial torsion serve to increase the child's angle of toe-out. Cadence is very high for infants to compensate for all of the other constraints.

6. Muscle strength

a. Answer refers to individual lab groups.

b. Extensor strength is essential for postural support. The strength develops gradually over the first year of life.

7. Motor control

Selective control over lower extremity muscles is necessary to enable the smooth shift in COG that occurs during gait. Muscles around each joint must be able to meet the demands of the ground reaction forces to maximize inertial forces and maintain forward momentum. Without selective control, a person can still stand and walk using the primitive flexion and extension patterns but the gait lacks the subtle mechanisms that absorb shock, conserve energy, and enable efficient forward progression.

8. a. Optic flow is the changing visual information received by the eye as it moves from one place to another.

b. Children use visual information for balance in an upright posture. While normal children also receive vestibular and proprioceptive input, the visual system seems to dominate. As individuals mature, they become less dominated by visual cues. Adult gait readily uses proprioceptive and vestibular input for balance. How did you do walking through the obstacle course blindfolded? If your gait pattern changed after you were blindfolded, you have evidence of the visual contributions to gait. If you could still maintain your balance and negotiate the course after being blindfolded, you realize the input of the proprioceptive and vestibular systems.

9. a. Smiles, words of encouragement, offering toys and food, interesting sounds and colorful objects to get their attention.

b. It seems that a positive, supportive environment encourages normal development while a negative, stressful environment inhibits and retards normal development. What ideas do you have to promote a positive, supportive environment for your patients?

Part 3. Parental Handling and Influences

1. Handling techniques that increase muscle tone and encourage the upright postures of sitting, standing, and walking involve placing the child in position, bouncing the child in position, providing unpredictable postural support while using encouraging verbal support, and using other children as role models for the desired behavior.

2. Balinese parents in the Mead and MacGregor (1951) study wanted their children to be lithe and graceful so they could do the traditional Balinese forms of dance.

3. The developmental sequence seen in the United States usually involves the following progression: quadripedal posture, belly crawling, creeping, cruising, standing, walking, and finally squatting. The children in the Mead and MacGregor study did very little creeping. They were either carried, held, or placed in a sitting position. Their developmental sequence involved: *frogging*, a quadripedal position with extreme hip external rotation, flexion, and abduction (reinforced by hours of being carried in this position on people's hips), and then bear-creeping simultaneously with cruising, squatting, and standing. Movement patterns in the Balinese children included spinal hyperextension, limb extension with external rotation, eversion, and ulnar grasp. A third difference was body posture including low tone, decreased joint synchrony, increased joint flexibility, body asymmetry, and a disassociation of the body parts. Mead and MacGregor attributed the children's passivity and flaccid postures to the fact that their parents and caretakers were constantly handling, holding, and carrying them. The combined effect of all of these factors resulted in a delay in independent ambulation.

Part 4. Early Gait Patterns

Section A

First Steps

1. A new walker uses high guard, a flat-footed initial contact, lack of knee flexion during midstance, a decreased step and stride length, an increased stance time, decreased single limb support, decreased velocity, and increased cadence.

2. Answer refers to individual lab groups.

Section B

Gait Patterns in Childhood

1. Heel strike—increases from footflat contact to a real heel strike.

2. Maximal knee flexion during stance—increases from 0° to 5° at age 2.

3. Arm swing—goes from high guard at 12 months to a reciprocal arm swing at age 4.

4. Step length—lengthens through childhood; mature pattern seen by age 7.

5. Stride length—lengthens through childhood; mature pattern seen by age 7.

6. Percentage stance time—decreases through childhood; mature pattern seen by age 7.

7. Single limb support—increases through childhood; mature pattern seen by age 7.

8. Cadence—decreases through childhood, with main reduction between ages 1 and 2.

9. Velocity—increases through childhood; mature pattern seen by age 7; rate of increase declines from age 4 to 7.

Part 5. Gait and Age

1. Velocity: decreases.

2. Step length: decreases.

3. Stride length: decreases.

4. Width of BOS: increases.

5. Angle of toe-out: increases.

6. Stance phase: increases.

7. Swing phase: decreases.

8. Double limb support: increases.

9. Vertical displacement of COG: decreases.

10. Lateral displacement of COG: may increase with increased width of BOS.

11. Arm swing: decreases.

12. Initial contact: decreased shock absorption.

13. Joint ranges of motion: decreases.

14. Joint synchrony: decreased ability to selectively control hip and knee movements.

15. Muscle strength: decreases.

16. Muscle activation patterns: increased coactivation, may have stiffness.

17. Basal metabolic rate: decreases approximately 2% during every decade of adulthood.

18. Maximal aerobic capacity (VO_2 max): decreases after approximately 20 years of age.

19. Postural control: decreases.

20. Sensory input: decreases.

21. Both the infant walkers and the older walkers show the following similarities in their gait characteristics: reduced step length, reduced velocity, decreased period of single limb support, increased duration of double limb support, increased width of BOS, increased toe-out, increased coactivation of agonist and antagonist muscles, and increased joint synchrony. Both the infants and the older walkers have problems with balance. The similarities seen in their gait characteristics are strategies for increasing stability. The reasons for balance problems in each group reflect very different causes.

Part 6. The Effect of Gender

1. VO_2 max: 15% to 20% greater in men than women.

2. Basal metabolic rate: 5% to 10% greater in men than women.

3. Energy expenditure: greater in men than women.

4. Step length: longer in men than women, though some of this is culturally conditioned.

5. Stride length: longer in men than women, though some of this is culturally conditioned.

6. Velocity: men are 5% faster than women; men average 85 m/min; women average 77 m/min.

7. Cadence: women have a greater cadence than men; women take 117 steps/min; men average 111 steps/min.

Part 7. The Kinesics of Gait

Section A

Age, Sex, and Emotional State

Answers refer to individual lab groups.

Section B

Sociocultural Factors in Gait

1. Depressed people, such as captives or conquered people.

2. Gait of children educated in a French Catholic convent school in the 1930's.

3. Maori gait.

4. An ancient Greek warrior.

5. Gait of an ancient Greek noblewoman.

6. Seaboard Algonkian warriors.

7. James Baldwin likened this gait to that of a "Harlem hipster."

Part 8. Thought Questions

Many answers to these questions are possible. The questions are provided for your thoughtful consideration.

Chapter 7
Pathological Gait and Clinical Examples
Part 1. Spastic Cerebral Palsy—Diplegia and Quadriplegia

Section A

Movement Experiments With Characteristic Gait Patterns

Answers refer to individual lab groups.

Section B

Pathokinematics in the Gait of People With Spastic Cerebral Palsy

Answers to Figure 7-1B-1.

1. Ankle—initial contact (IC): forefoot contact that constitutes excessive plantarflexion. Loading response (LR): ankle dorsiflexes to neutral. Midstance (MSt): dorsiflexion continues, premature heel rise occurs with the knee flexed, creating an unstable situation; the ankle continues to dorsiflex. Terminal stance (TSt): excessive heel rise and a related rapid ankle plantarflexion. Preswing (PSw): high heel rise with slight ankle dorsiflexion.

   Swing—brief toe drag, the ankle dorsiflexes slowly and achieves a nearly neutral position by the end of swing.

   Knee—excessive flexion seen throughout the gait cycle; less knee flexion is seen during MSt but an unstable situation develops during TSt as knee flexion increases with early heel rise. In swing, knee flexion persists, interfering with tibial advancement in midswing (MSw) and resulting in inadequate knee extension during terminal swing (TSw).

   Hip—within normal limits throughout the gait cycle.

   Thigh—throughout the gait cycle the thigh is excessively flexed; it fails to achieve a trailing position in TSt. PSw: thigh advancement as body weight is transferred to contralateral limb. During swing, excessive flexion continues (but at a rate slower than normal); this causes a shortened step length.

   Pelvis—TSt: posterio-lateral pelvic drop; continuous posterior pelvic tilt throughout the gait cycle.

2. Crouch gait.

3. The patient is hyperpronating through the transverse tarsal joint.

4. Obliterates the heel rocker mechanism but provides some stability in early stance.

5. Mostly due to excessive knee flexion.

6. Closed-chain reaction to position of the foot, ankle, and knee.

7. Hip range of motion is modified by posterior tilt of the pelvis.

Section C

Pathokinetics in the Gait of People With Spastic Cerebral Palsy

1. Three.

2. Figures 7-1C-1 and 7-1C-2 show activation of gracilis, semimembranosus, and the long head of biceps femoris from IC through MSt and from late TSt through initial swing (ISw) a with low level of activity continuing through the end of swing. The biceps femoris short head is also active from late TSt through ISw. Iliacus and gracilis are active throughout swing; rectus femoris (beginning in MSw and TSw), and adductor longus (in TSw). Adductor longus continues through TSt. Rectus femoris and the vastus intermedius are active throughout the gait cycle.

3. At the knee, abnormal coactivation flexion synergy is seen from IC through MSt and from late TSt through ISw involving gracilis, semimembranosus, and the long head of the biceps femoris. The biceps femoris short head is involved in the latter pattern.

   The rectus femoris and vastus intermedius have prolonged activity throughout the gait cycle but this is useful during stance to help stabilize the flexed knee. The adductor longus is abnormally active during stance but this is also useful because it assists with hip flexion at TSw to lengthen the step a bit.

Section D

The main problems are excessive knee flexion, ankle plantarflexion contracture, and inappropriate activity of the hamstrings, rectus femoris, adductor longus, and vastus intermedius. The knee flexion during stance destabilizes the limb and necessitates prolonged quadriceps activity. The ankle plantarflexion contracture interferes with the heel and rocker mechanisms impeding forward progression and energy conservation. Many treatment strategies are reasonable. Any approach to lessen knee flexion is appropriate and may include: passive stretch, myofascial release, serial casting, plantarflexion, or similar techniques. Exercises to improve motor and orthotic management of the foot and ankle are also indicated.

Part 2. Gait of a Person With a Transtibial Amputation

Section A

General Concepts

1. Sensation

    a. Proprioception and kinesthesia so you will know where your limbs are in space; light touch so you can tell if anything is causing a laceration or irritation; vestibular input to help you maintain your dynamic balance; visual input to help you avoid obstacles and maintain your balance.

    b. Visual input compensating for proprioceptive input as patients watch instead of feel where they are placing their prosthetic feet; auditory input compensating for proprioceptive input as patients listen for the "click" of the prosthetic knee locking into extension during TSw or the sound of the prosthetic heel contacting the ground at IC; light touch of the socket around the stump to compensate for proprioception in the absent limb.

2. The cushion heel compresses during IC and LR to absorb shock and enable footflat without excessively advancing the shin and destabilizing the knee. Compression of the solid ankle-cushion heel (SACH) permits some adaptation to uneven surfaces and a simulation of the heel rocker to maintain forward progression and energy conservation. The SACH foot does not permit ankle motion so no ankle rocker mechanism is possible. The rubber forefoot substitutes for the forefoot rocker and helps maintain forward momentum; however, good control at the knee is necessary for stability during TSt.

3. The ankle strategy involves plantarflexion and forward sway that occurs after a forward perturbation. Dorsiflexion with a backward sway occurs following a backward perturbation. Strategies that people with prosthetic legs can use to maintain dynamic equilibrium will probably involve using hip strategies instead of ankle strategies.

Section B

Pathokinematics

Answers to Figure 7-2B-1.

Ankle—LR through MSt: slightly increased dorsiflexion. TSt: excessive dorsiflexion. PSw: inadequate plantarflexion which comes to neutral as the limb is unloaded. Swing: ankle in neutral.

Knee—hyperextension at 40% of the gait cycle and at the end of TSw; increased knee flexion from PSw through MSw.

Hip—generally within normal limits; slight increase in hip flexion during ISw and MSw.

Thigh—LR through MSt: forward inclination of the thigh (reduced flexion). MSw through TSw: increased forward inclination.

Pelvis—continuous anterior tilt.

1. Helps displace the ground reaction force vector anteriorly to help stabilize the limb during stance.

2. Enables the knee to fully extend and permits good forward progression.

3. The prosthetic foot is permitting excessive dorsiflexion (or inadequate plantarflexion) to help maintain forward progression. The prosthetic ankle dorsiflexion is passive. As the foot is unweighted, the prosthetic ankle returns to neutral where it remains throughout swing.

Section C

Pathokinetics

1. Three.

2. The patient has activation of the gluteus maximus, the hamstring muscles, and the vastus longus during the end of swing phase and at the beginning of stance. Rectus femoris shows a burst of activity in TSt and PSw.

3. The patient has increased activation and intensity of gluteus maximus and hamstring muscles to extend the limb and stabilize the thigh in TSw in preparation for weight-bearing at IC. Quadriceps (vastus longus) action is prolonged to control the increased knee flexion. Rectus femoris shows a burst of activity in TSt and PSw to control the excessive knee flexion.

Section D

The patient has hyperextension of the knee in TSt and at the end of TSw and excessive knee flexion in PSw and ISw. The prosthetic ankle is excessively dorsiflexed in TSt and in neutral throughout swing. The pelvis is in a continual anterior pelvic tilt. The major muscles show an increase in intensity and duration. These are reasonable accommodations for using a prosthetic limb. If the patient is not reporting any problems, I do not modify the limb. If the patient is having difficulty, I speak with the prosthetist about modifying the ankle.

Part 3. Spinal Cord Injury

Section A

General Concepts

1. a. T4-6—the patient has use of both upper extremities, latissimus dorsi, upper intercostals and upper erector spinae. The patient will need orthotic devices for standing and gait. The patient is independent in transfers and is a physiological ambulator. A wheelchair is necessary for household and community mobility.

   b. T_{9-12}—the patient has the use of the intercostals, erector spinae, and the abdominal muscles; with orthoses, the patient may achieve household ambulation and limited stair climbing. A wheelchair is necessary for community mobility.

   c. L_{1-4}—the patient has the use of the hip flexors, the adductors, and knee extension. The patient can be a household ambulator with orthoses, but a wheelchair is necessary for community mobility.

   d. L_5-S_1—the patient has the use of all or most of the hip muscles, knee extension, weak knee flexion, and partial use of the ankle dorsiflexors and plantarflexors. Community mobility is reasonable with ankle-foot orthoses. The patient may want to use a wheelchair for convenience.

2. Joint contractures—the presence of joint contractures may set the patient back one functional level.

3. Degree of spasticity—severe spasticity may hinder the patient's functional level.

4. Body weight—heavier patients require more energy for mobility and have more difficulty.

5. Upper body strength, fitness, and general athleticism—the better shape the patient was in before the injury the better off he or she is in rehabilitation.

6. Sensation—intact sensation is important for functional gait; you need to know where your limbs are in space and whether they are safe from abrasions and injury.

7. Age—younger patients generally do better that older patients.

8. General health—healthier patients do better than people with complex medical problems.

9. Psychological factors and motivation—highly motivated people do better than others; people who are depressed do not do as well.

10. Sociocultural factors including home and community support systems—clearly supportive families and social networks are best.

Section B

Pathokinematics

Answers to Figure 7-3B-1.

Ankle—IC: The ankle is plantarflexed. LR through PSw: The ankle dorsiflexes throughout stance, and there is delayed heel rise during TSt. The ankle is excessively dorsiflexed at PSw. Swing: no plantarflexion is seen in ISw, and the ankle remains dorsiflexed throughout swing.

Knee—IC: within normal limits (WNL). LR: inadequate knee flexion. MSt: WNL. TSt: inadequate knee flexion at the end when heel rise should occur. PSw: inadequate knee flexion. Swing: inadequate knee flexion.

Hip—inadequate knee flexion of the contralateral limb during PSw puts the foot of the reference limb too high in TSw. In order to contact the ground at IC, the reference hip does not fully flex. This inadequate hip flexion remains through LR and then the hip extends excessively until TSt. During swing, increased hip flexion helps clear the foot in ISw but inadequate hip flexion is seen in MSw and TSw in response to the contralateral limb.

Thigh—WNL.

Pelvis—maintains an anterior pelvic tilt that increases during early swing.

1. The anterior pelvic tilt helps the trunk maintain an upright position and compensates for the limited motion seen at the hip.

2. Major deviations are seen at the knee and the ankle. Knee extension gives the patient a stable limb for weight-bearing. Ankle dorsiflexion in late stance provides a substitution for the forefoot rocker and permits better foot clearance during swing.

3. In TSt the right thigh is extended, the right hip is hyperextended, the right knee is extended, and the right ankle is dorsiflexed. This positions the body above the stance limb (instead of in advance of it) and functions to shorten the step length.

Section C

Pathokinesics

1. The electromyogram (EMG) tracings are notable for the intense activity represented in the vasti muscles with very little activity evident in any of the other groups. Hamstrings do show some very low intensity activity during IC but the effect is overridden by the vasti.

2. These are very abnormal tracings (Figures 7-3C-1 and 7-3C-2). The normal vasti activity is from IC through early MSt and during TSw. This patient has continuous activity throughout the gait cycle. Rectus femoris is normally active during PSw and ISw but in this patient rectus femoris activity is almost absent. Hamstring activity is also abnormal. They should be active during IC and at the end of swing but their activation in this patient is very low throughout the gait cycle.

Section D

The patient has a stiff knee gait with the knee extended and held in position by excessive activation of the vasti. Excessive ankle dorsiflexion provides a substitution for the forefoot rocker and permits better foot clearance during swing. The anterior pelvic tilt helps the trunk maintain an upright position and compensates for the limited motion seen at the hip. I would try some functional electrical stimulation to the hamstrings to see if more knee flexion is possible and experiment with ankle foot orthoses to simulate the foot and ankle mechanisms and achieve better forward progression. If possible, it would be nice to strengthen the knee flexors and the ankle plantarflexors.

Part 4. Peripheral Neuropathy

Section A

General Background

1. a. Metabolic disorder—diabetes.

b. Trauma—crush, compression, stretch (traction), inflammatory, and entrapment: gunshot, stabbing, thoracic outlet syndrome, carpal tunnel syndrome, tarsal tunnel syndrome, etc.

c. Chemical toxicity—lead, arsenic.

2. Chart comparing peripheral nerves to motor neurons.

Nerve and Neuron Table

	Peripheral Nerve	Upper Motor Neuron
a. Ability to regenerate	yes	no
b. Muscle changes after a complete lesion	atrophy, weakness, low tone	weakness, increased tone
c. Sensation when nerve is compressed	numbness and paresthesia	painless or paresthesia
d. Sensation after compression is released	"pins and needles," "release phenomenon"	pain free
e. Sensory distribution	extra-segmental; peripheral nerve distribution	segmental

Answer Figure 7-4A-1.

Section B

Pathokinematics

1. Common peroneal nerve (Answer to Figure 7-4B-1).

2. The foot would tend to have a forefoot contact at IC and excessively supinate from midstance through the end of stance phase. Toes will drag during swing. The patient may trip over or have difficulty clearing the toes during swing phase.

3. Excessive ankle plantarflexion IC through LR; excessive plantarflexion through stance phase and toe drag or excessive plantarflexion during swing.

Section C

1. The foot would tend to hypersupinate from midstance through end of stance phase because the gastrocsoleus group is working and pronators (which normally fire to eccentrically control supination) are absent. The toes will drag during swing. The tibialis anterior and all of the toe extensors are weak or absent.

2. Because of sensory deficit, the patient may not know where the foot is in space and may twist the ankle or trip over the toes.

Section D

Summary

Lack of sensation and impaired motor function put this patient at high risk for injuring the foot and ankle. The treatment plan needs to recognize this risk and offer some protection. Orthotic management and patient education are indicated.

Part 5. Adult Hemiplegia

Section A

General Concepts

1. An occlusion of the left middle cerebral artery as it leaves the Circle of Willis will compromise blood supply to the internal capsule, resulting in damage to the descending tracts from the precentral gyrus in the central fissure and to most medial areas of the cortex. Looking at the motor homunculus, you will see that this area sends descending innervation to the entire right lower extremity, right upper extremity, and right side of the trunk, and the right side of the face, the mouth, and the tongue. All of these parts of the body will be affected.

2. The patient may be flaccid immediately after the stroke but with a recovery period, increased tone (spasticity) may develop.

3. a. Drop foot—weakness of the ankle dorsiflexors, inability to selectively recruit dorsiflexor muscles, and the effect of the primitive extension pattern.

   b. Genu recurvatum—extensor (quadriceps) spasticity, the effect of the primitive extension pattern, and an inability to selectively recruit knee flexors during stance.

c. Excessive hindfoot supination—extensor (gastrocnemius) spasticity and the effect of the primitive extension pattern.

d. Inadequate knee flexion—extensor (quadriceps and gastrocnemius) spasticity and the effect of the primitive extension pattern.

Section B

Pathokinematics

Answers to Figure 7-5B-1.

Ankle—fixed in plantarflexion throughout gait cycle; normal rocker mechanisms are absent.

Knee—hyperextended throughout stance, especially in MSt; the knee flexes in ISw and then returns to hyperextension. The patient is using a pass-retract maneuver during TSw to achieve full knee extension for IC. Normally, the knee should flex in IC through LR, extend during MSt and TSt, flex during PSw and ISw, and extend during MSw and TSw.

1. Here are two strategies: The patient can laterally lean to the opposite side, or the patient can retract (backwardly rotate) the pelvis on the hemiplegic side and use the hip adductors to assist the hip flexors in advancing the limb.

2. The hemiplegic hip can be expected to have limited flexion and the pelvis may drop on the nonhemiplegic side due to weakness in the gluteus medius and may have an anterior pelvic tilt to help maintain the torso in an upright position.

3. The contralateral limb may have a longer stance duration than the hemiplegic limb and a shorter step length. The contralateral limb may have a low heel strike or footflat contact at the beginning of stance and low heel rise or prolonged foot contact at the end of stance. Double limb support may be increased.

Section C

Pathokinetics

Answers to Figures 7-5C-1 and 7-5C-2.

1. The EMG shows minimal activation of soleus and gastrocnemius. This seems surprising because the ankle is continuously held in plantarflexion. Plantarflexion of the joint without activation of the plantarflexor muscles indicates a contracture. Strong continuous activation is seen in the tibialis anterior, the flexor hallucis longus, and the peroneus longus. The tibialis anterior may be trying to prevent toe drag during swing and assists with tibial advance during stance. The flexor hallucis longus and peroneus longus may also be trying to act on the tibia during stance.

2. The EMG tracings are clearly abnormal (Figures 7-5C-1 and 7-5C-2). Ankle plantarflexors should only be active from LR through TSt. The tibialis anterior should be active from IC through LR and from PSw through swing phase.

Section D

The patient has a severe plantarflexor contracture at the ankle and severe recurvatum at the knee. The EMG shows minimal activation of the soleus and the gastrocneumius with continuous activation seen in the tibialis anterior, the flexor hallucis longus, and the peroneus longus. This indicates a lack of selective muscle control but there is no evidence of the primitive flexion and extension patterns.

Part 6. Gait Deviations in People With Parkinson's Disease

1. The lesion is in the substantia nigra of the basal ganglia.

2. Characteristic signs and symptoms of Parkinson's disease include difficulty initiating movement, difficulty maintaining postural control, *pill-rolling* tremor at rest, cog-wheel rigidity, and a mask-like face.

3. Parkinsonian gait has been described as shuffling with a stooped posture. Specific gait deviations include reduced velocity; a decreased, often asymmetric step length; an increased cadence; flat foot or forefoot contact at IC; forward trunk lean; decreased trunk counter-rotation with the pelvis; decreased or absent arm swing; decreased swing phases; and increased periods of double limb support. Normal postural control mechanisms are absent or depressed. The shuffling gait pattern is seen in the early stages of Parkinson's disease. People in the late stages of the disease may demonstrate a festinating or propulsive gait pattern in which the body leans forward and the cadence increases as the person's steps try to catch up with the forward falling center of gravity. Gait deviations show a large variation between people.

4. Joint excursions for all of the joints of the locomotor unit are reduced resulting in an ankle joint with reduced plantarflexion during LR and the end of stance; reduced dorsiflexion during TSt; inadequate knee extension in MSt through TSt and at the end of TSw; inadequate knee flexion during PSw, ISw, and MSw; and decreased hip flexion at the beginning of stance and during swing with decreased hip extension during TSt.

5. The activation patterns of the muscles in people with Parkinson's disease may be similar to normal people but the intensity of the muscle activation is increased. No relaxation periods may exist so there may be continuous coactivation between agonist and antagonist groups resulting in muscle rigidity.

6. Parkinsonian gait has been described as a stooped, shuffling, or festinating gait. The person has decreased movement in the trunk, arms, and lower extremities. Velocity is slowed, though cadence may actually increase. Postural control is decreased and people have a tendency to fall forward. Continuous coactivation between agonist and antagonist groups is seen resulting in muscle rigidity. Treatment includes helping patients maintain their joint mobility, improve their postural control, and maintain as normal a gait pattern as possible. Knutsson and Martensson (1986) reported that one researcher found that better postural control can be achieved if the patient is rocked from side to side. Klawans, Goetz, and Tanner (1988) described improved gait if patients have obstacles on the floor that they have to step over.

Part 7. Gait Deviations in People With Down Syndrome

1. Nondisjunction—unequal cell division that occurs during oogenesis and spermatogenesis.
Translocation—a transfer of genetic material from one chromosome to another.
Mosaicism—a form of nondisjunction that occurs after fertilization.

2. People with Down syndrome characteristically have low tone, short stature, mental retardation, developmental delay, a small nose and low nasal bridge, short and stubby fingers, almond-shaped eyes, a simian crease on their palms, and heart defects.

3. Parker and Bronks (1980) described the gait of six children with Down syndrome who were all approximately 7 years old. These children had relatively longer stance and shorter swing phases with a wider BOS and increased toe-out. The children tended to have a flat-foot contact with decreased ankle and knee excursions throughout the gait cycle. Foot contact at the end of stance was often prolonged. Hip extension during TSt was significantly reduced when compared with normal adults. Motion in the arms was highly variable but increased wrist flexion throughout the gait cycle was characteristic of the children in this study. The authors concluded that the children in their study had gait patterns closely resembling the immature patterns of new walkers but that considerable variation existed between their subjects.

4. Flat-foot contact, prolonged foot contact in PSw, decreased ankle and knee excursions throughout the gait cycle, and reduced hip extension during TSt are some of the characteristic kinematic features.

5. Low muscle tone and the inefficiency of the gait pattern suggests that increased muscle activation is required. Further research is needed to support this hypothesis.

6. Down syndrome gait patterns include relatively longer stance and shorter swing phases with a wider BOS and increased toe-out, low muscle tone, flat-foot contact, prolonged foot contact in PSw decreased ankle and knee excursions throughout the gait cycle, reduced hip extension during TSt, and increased wrist flexion throughout the gait cycle. Reasonable treatment approaches include improving static and dynamic balance, closed-chain exercises to improve strength and endurance of the foot and ankle muscles, exercises to improve single limb support, and exercises to improve postural control.

Part 8. Center of Gravity Displacement Problems

This part is a synthesis of material presented in earlier chapters. Refer to answers from appropriate chapters.

References

Chapter 1

Elftman, H. (1954). The functional structure of the lower limb. In P. E. Klopsteg & P. D. Wilson (Eds.), *Human limbs and their substitutes* (pp. 411-436). New York: McGraw-Hill Book Co.

Perry, J. (1992). *Gait analysis: Normal and pathological function*. Thorofare, NJ: SLACK Incorporated.

Chapter 2

Baker, H. H., Bruckner, J. S., & Langdon, J. H. (1992). Estimating ankle rotational constraints from anatomic structure. *Visualization in Biomedical Computing Proc SPIE, 1808*, 422-432.

Engsberg, J. R. (1987). A biomechanical analysis of the talocalcaneal joint-in vitro. *Journal of Biomechanics. 20*(4), 429-442.

Inman, V. T., & Mann, R. A. (1973). Biomechanics of the foot and ankle. In V. T. Inman (Ed.), *DuVries' surgery of the foot* (2nd ed.). St. Louis, MO: C.V. Mosby Co.

Isman, R. E., & Inman, V. T. (1969). Anthropometric studies of the human foot and ankle. *Bull. of Pros. Res., 10*, 97-129.

Kirby, K. A. (1989). Rotational equilibrium across the subtalar joint axis. *Journal of the American Podiatric Medical Association, 79*(1), 1-14.

Laidlaw, P. P. (1904). The varieties of the os calcis. *Journal of Anatomy, 38*, 133-143.

Manter, J. T. (1941). Movements of the subtalar and transverse tarsal joints. *Anatomical Record, 80*, 397-410.

Perry, J. (1992). *Gait analysis: Normal and pathological function*. Thorofare, NJ: SLACK Incorporated.

Root, M. L., Weed, J. H., Sgarlato, T. E., & Bluth, D. R. (1966). Axis motion of the subtalar joint: an anatomical study. *Journal of the American Podiatry Association, 56*, 149-155.

Siegler, S., Chen, J., & Schneck, C. D. (1988). The three-dimensional kinematics and flexibility characteristics of the human ankle and the subtalar joints—part 1: kinematics. *Journal of Biomechanical Engineering, 110*, 364-373.

Chapter 3

Kettlecamp, D. B., Johnson, R. J., Smidt, G. L., Chao, E. Y., & Walker, M. (1970). An electrogoniometric study of knee motion in normal gait. *Journal of Bone Joint Surg, 52A*(4), 775-790.

Chapter 4

Murray, M. P., Drought, A. B., & Kory, R. C. (1964). Walking patterns in normal men. *J Bone Joint Surg, 46(2A)*, 335-360.

Murray, M. P., Kory, R. C., & Sepic, S. B. (1970). Walking patterns in normal women. *Arch Phys Med Rehab, 51*, 637-650.

Chapter 5

Elftman, H. (1954). The functional structure of the lower limb. In P. E. Klopsteg & P. D. Wilson (Eds.), *Human limbs and their substitutes* (pp. 411-436). New York: McGraw-Hill Book Co.

Chapter 6

Baldwin, J. (1965). Sonny's blues. In *Going to meet the man* (p. 130). New York: Dial Press.

Birdwhistell, R. L. (1970). *Kinesics and context: Essays on body motion communication*. Philadelphia: University of Pennsylvania Press.

Bremmer, J. (1991). Walking, standing and sitting in ancient Greek culture. In J. Bremmer & H. Roodenburg (Eds.), *A cultural history of gesture* (pp. 16-23). Ithaca, NY: Cornell University Press.

Flinn, M. V., & England, B. G. (1997). Social economics of childhood glucocorticoid stress response and health. *American Journal of Physical Anthropology, 102*, 33-53.

Gardner, L. I. (1973). Deprivation dwarfism. In W. T. Greenough (Ed.), *The nature and nuture of behavior: Developmental psychobiology* (pp. 101-107). San Francisco: W. H. Freeman & Co.

Gruber, M. I. (1980). *Aspects of non-verbal communication in the ancient Near East* (p. 127). Rome: Biblical Institute Press.

Hopkins, B., & Westra, T. (1988). Maternal handling and motor development: An intercultural study. *Genetic, Socical, and General Psychology Monographs, 114,* 377-408.

Konner, M. (1976). Maternal care, infant behavior and development among the !Kung. In R. B. Lee & I. DeVore (Eds.), *Kalahari hunter-gatherers: Studies of the !Kung San and their neighbors* (pp. 218-245). Cambridge, MA: Harvard University Press.

Lee, S. (1995). *Impressions created by gait: The effect of childlike physical attributes on trait inference.* Unpublished doctoral thesis. Seoul, Korea: Yonsei University Psychology Dept.

Maus, M. (1973). Les techniques du corps. In B. Brewster (Trans.), Techniques of the body. *Economy and Society, 2*(1), 70-88.

Mead, M., & Macgregor, F. C. (1951). *Growth and culture: A photographic study of Balinese childhood.* New York: G. P. Putnam's Sons.

Montepare, J. M., & Zebrowitz, L. A. (1993). A cross-cultural comparison of impressions created by age-related variation in gait. *Journal of Nonverbal Behavior, 17,* 55-68.

Montepare, J. M., & Zebrowitz-McArthur, L. (1988). Impressions of people created by age-related qualities of their gaits. *Journal of Personality and Social Psychology, 55,* 547-556.

Nashner, L. M. (1977). Fixed patterns of rapid postural response among leg muscles during stance. *Experimental Brain Research, 30,* 13-24.

Nashner, L., & Woollacott, M. (1979). The organization of rapid postural adjustments of standing humans: An experimental-conceptual model. In R. E. Talbott & D. R. Humphrey (Eds.), *Posture and movement* (pp. 243-257). New York: Raven Press.

Perry, J. (1992). *Gait analysis: Normal and pathological function.* Thorofare, NJ: SLACK Incorporated.

Super, C. M. (1976). Environmental effects on motor development: The case of "African infant precocity." *Developmental Medicine and Child Neurology, 18,* 561-567.

Thelen, E., Ulrich, B. D., & Jensen, J. L. (1989). The developmental origins of locomotion. In M. H. Woollacott & A. Shumway-Cook (Eds.), *Development of posture and gait across the life span* (pp. 25-47). Columbia: University of South Carolina.

Underhill, R. M. (1953). *Red Man's America: A history of Indians in the United States* (p. 70). Chicago, IL: University of Chicago Press.

Chapter 7

Gage, J. R. (1991). *Gait analysis in cerebral palsy.* London: MacKeith Press.

Horak, F., & Nashner, L. (1986). Central programming of postural movements: Adaptations to altered support surface configurations. *Journal of Neurophysiology, 55,* 1369-1381.

Nashner, L. M. (1977). Fixed patterns of rapid postural response among leg muscles during stance. *Experimental Brain Research, 30,* 13-24.

Nashner, L., & Woollacott, M. (1979). The organization of rapid postural adjustments of standing humans: An experimental-conceptual model. In R. E. Talbott & D. R. Humphrey (Eds.), *Posture and movement* (pp. 243-257). New York: Raven Press.

Perry, J. (1992). *Gait analysis: Normal and pathological function.* Thorofare, NJ: SLACK Incorporated.

Shumway-Cook, A., & Woollacott, M. H. (1995). *Motor control theory and practical applications* (pp. 308-310). Baltimore: Williams & Wilkins.

Recommended Reading

Chapter 1

Hoppenfeld, S. (1976). *Physical examination of the spine and extremities.* New York: Appleton-Century-Crofts.

Lower limb orthotics. (1981). New York: New York University Post-Graduate Medical School.

Norkin, C. C., & Levangie, P. K. (1992). *Joint structure and function: A comprehensive analysis* (2nd ed.). Philadelphia: F. A. Davis Co, 1992.

Chapter 2

Bojsen-Moller, F., & Lamoreux, L. (1979). Significance of free dorsiflexion of the toes in walking. *Acta Orthopaedica Scandinavica, 50,* 471-479.

Bordelon, R. L. (1983). Hypermobile flatfeet in children. *Clinical Orthopaedics and Related Research, 181*, 7-14.

Bruckner, J. S. (1987). Variations in the human subtalar joint. *Journal of Orthopedic and Sports Physical Therapy, 8*, 489-494.

Bunning, P. S. C. (1964). Some observations on the West African calcaneus and associated talo-calcaneal interosseous ligamentous apparatus. *American Journal of Physical Anthropology, 22*, 467-472.

Bunning, P. S. C., & Barnett, C. H. (1965). A comparision of adult and foetal talocalcaneal articulations. *Journal of Anatomy, 99*, 71-75.

Bunning, P. S. C., & Barnett, C. H. (1963). Variations in the talocalcaneal articulation. *Journal of Anatomy, 97*, 643.

Campos, F. F., & Pellico, L. G. (1989). Talar articular facets in human calcanei. *Acta Anatomica, 134*, 124-127.

Cyriax, J., & Cyriax, P. (1983). *Illustrated manual of orthopaedic medicine* (pp. 111-130). London: Butterworths.

Donatelli, R. A. (1987). Abnormal biomechanics of the foot and ankle. *Journal of Orthopedic and Sports Physical Therapy, 9*(1), 11-16.

Donatelli, R. A. (1990). *The biomechanics of the foot and ankle* (2nd ed., pp. 3-72, 90-123). Philadelphia, PA: F. A. Davis Co.

El-Eishi, H. (1974). Variations in the talar articular facets in Egyptian calcanei. *Acta Anatomica, 89*, 134-138.

Finnegan, M., & Faust, M. W. (1974). *Bibliography of human and nonhuman non-metric variation*. Res. Reports No. 4. Amherst, MA: University of Massachusetts.

Gould, N. (1983). Evaluation of hyperpronation and pes planus in adults. *Clinical Orthopaedics and Related Research, 181*, 37-45.

Gray, G. W. (1984). *When the feet hit the ground everything changes: Program outline and prepared notes*. Toledo, OH: American Physical Rehabilitation Network.

Gupta, S. C., Gupta, C. D., & Arora, A. K. (1977). Pattern of talar articular facets in Indian calcanei. *Journal of Anatomy, 124*(3), 651-655.

Hicks, J. H. (1954). The foot as a support. *Acta Anatomica, 25*, 34-45.

Hicks, J. H. (1953). The mechanic of the foot I: The joints. *Journal of Anatomy, 87*, 345-357.

Hicks, J. H. (1954). The mechanic of the foot II The plantar aponeurosis and the arch. *Journal of Anatomy, 88*, 25-30.

Hoppenfeld, S. (1976). *Physical examination of the spine and extremities*. New York: Appleton-Century-Crofts.

Hrdlicka, A. (1916). Physical anthropology of the Lenape or Delawares and of the eastern Indians in general. *BAE Bull, 62*, 96-97.

Inman, V. T. (1974). Hallux valgus: A review of etiologic factors. *Orthopedic Clinics of North America, 5*(1), 59-67.

Kendall, F. P., McCreary, E. K., & Provance, P. G. (1993). *Muscles: Testing and function* (4th ed.). Baltimore: Williams & Wilkins.

Magee, D. J. (1992). *Orthopedic physical assessment* (pp. 448-515). Philadelphia: W. B. Saunders Co.

McPoil, T. G., & Brocato, R. S. (1990). The foot and ankle: Biomechanical evaluation and treatment. In J. A. Gould (Ed.), *Orthopaedic and sports physical therapy* (2nd ed., pp. 293-321). St. Louis, MO: C.V. Mosby Co.

Norkin, C. C., & Levangie, P. K. (1992). *Joint structure and function: A comprehensive analysis* (2nd ed.). Philadelphia: F. A. Davis Co.

Observational gait analysis (pp. 8-13, 34-38). (1993). Downey, CA: Los Amigos Research and Education Institute.

Powell, M. A., & Cantab, M. B. (1983). Pes planovalgus in children. *Clinical Orthopaedics and Related Research, 177*, 133-139.

Samilson, R. L., & Dillin, W. (1983). Cavus, cavovarus, and calcaneocavus. *Clin Orthop., 177*, 125-132.

Spencer, A. M. (1978). *Practical podiatric orthopedic procedures* (pp. 13-28). Cleveland, OH: Ohio College of Podiatric Medicine.

Tiberio, D. (1987). The effect of excessive subtalar joint pronation on patellofemoral mechanics: A theoretical model. *Journal of Orthopedic and Sports Physical Therapy, 9*(4), 160-165.

Tiberio, D. (1988). Pathomechanics of structural foot deformities. *Physical Therapy, 68*(12), 1840-1849.

Viladot, A., Lorenzo, J. C., Salazar, J., & Rodriguez, A. (1984). The subtalar joint: Embryology and morphology. *Foot and Ankle, 5*, 54-66.

Waller, J. F. (1980). Hindfoot and midfoot problems of the runner. In R. P. Mack (Ed.), *Symposium on the foot and leg in running sports* (pp. 64-72). St. Louis, MO: C.V. Mosby Co.

Chapter 3

Cyriax, J., & Cyriax, P. (1983). *Illustrated manual of orthopaedic medicine* (pp. 87-104). London: Butterworths.

Magee, DJ. (1992). *Orthopedic physical assessment* (pp. 372-447). Philadelphia, PA: W. B. Saunders.

Norkin, C. C., & Levangie, P. K. (1992). *Joint structure and function: A comprehensive analysis* (2nd ed.). Philadelphia: F. A. Davis Co.

Observational gait analysis (pp. 14-17, 40-43). (1993). Downey, CA: Los Amigos Research and Education Institute.

Perry, J. (1992). *Gait analysis: Normal and pathological function*. Thorofare, NJ: SLACK Incorporated.

Purtillo, D. T., & Purtillo, R. B. (1989). *A survey of human diseases* (2nd ed., pp. 535-536). Boston, MA: Little, Brown & Co.

Wallace, L. A., Mangine, R. E., & Malone, T. R. (1990). The knee. In J. A. Gould (Ed.), *Orthopaedic and sports physical therapy* (2nd ed., pp. 323-345). St. Louis, MO: C. V. Mosby Co.

Chapter 4

Batshaw, M. L., & Perret, Y. M. (1981). *Children with handicaps: A medical primer* (pp. 175-176). Baltimore: Paul H. Brookes.

Cyriax, J., & Cyriax, P. (1983). *Illustrated manual of orthopaedic medicine* (pp. 73-86). London: Butterworths.

Hunt, G. C. (1990). Examination of lower extremity dysfunction. In J. A. Gould (Ed.), *Orthopaedic and sports physical therapy* (2nd ed., pp. 395-421). St. Louis, MO: C. V. Mosby Co.

Magee, D. J. (1992). *Orthopedic physical assessment* (pp. 333-371). Philadelphia: W. B. Saunders.

Norkin, C. C., & Levangie, P. K. (1992). *Joint structure and function: A comprehensive analysis* (2nd ed.). Philadelphia, PA: F. A. Davis Co.

Observational gait analysis (pp. 18-20, 44-47). (1993). Downey, CA, Los Amigos Research and Education Institute.

Perry, J. (1992). *Gait analysis: Normal and pathological function*. Thorofare, NJ: SLACK Incorporated.

Purtillo, D. T., & Purtillo, R. B. (1989). *A survey of human diseases* (2nd ed., p. 535). Boston, MA: Little, Brown & Co.

Saudek, C. E. (1990). The hip. In J. A. Gould (Ed.), *Orthopaedic and sports physical therapy* (2nd ed., pp. 347-394). St. Louis, MO: C. V. Mosby Co.

Schmitz, T. J. (1994). Traumatic spinal cord injury. In S. B. O'Sullivan & T. J. Schmitz (Eds.), *Physical rehabilitation: Assessment and treatment* (3rd ed., pp. 533-575). Philadelphia: F. A. Davis Co.

Chapter 5

Hoppenfeld, S. (1976). *Physical examination of the spine and extremities*. New York: Appleton-Century-Crofts.

Hunt, G. C. (1990). Examination of lower extremity dysfunction. In J. A. Gould (Ed.), *Orthopaedic and sports physical therapy* (2nd ed., pp. 395-421). St. Louis, MO: C. V. Mosby Co.

Lower limb orthotics. (1981). New York: New York University Post-Graduate Medical School.

Norkin, C. C., & Levangie, P. K. (1992). *Joint structure and function: A comprehensive analysis* (2nd ed.). Philadelphia: F. A. Davis Co.

Observational gait analysis (pp. 18-20, 44-47). (1993). Downey, CA, Los Amigos Research and Education Institute.

Perry, J. (1992). *Gait analysis: Normal and pathological function*. Thorofare, NJ: SLACK Inc.

Schmitz, T. J. (1994). Traumatic spinal cord injury. In S. B. O'Sullivan & T. J. Schmitz (Eds.), *Physical rehabilitation: Assessment and treatment* (3rd ed., pp. 533-575). Philadelphia: F. A. Davis Co.

Trautman, P. (1995). Lower limb orthoses. In J. B. Redford, J. V. Basmajian, & P. Trautman (Eds.), *Orthotics: Clinical practice and rehabilitation technology* (pp. 13-53). New York: Churchill Livingstone.

Chapter 6

Alexander, R., Boehme, R., & Cupps, B. (1993). *Normal development of functional motor skills: The first year of life*. Tucson, AZ: Therapy Skill Builders.

Barnes, M. R., Crutchfield, C., & Heriza, C. (1978). *The neurophysiological basis of patient treatment: Vol. 2. Reflexes in motor development*. Morgantown, WV: Stokes Publishing Co.

Barnes, M. R., Crutchfield, C. A., Heriza, C. E., & Herdman, S. J. (1990). *Reflex and vestibular aspects of motor control, motor development and motor learning.* Atlanta, GA: Stokesville Publishing Co.

Bly, L. (1994). *Motor skills acquisition in the first year: An illustrated guide to normal development.* Tucson, AZ: Therapy Skill Builders.

Cutting, J. E., & Kozlowski, L. T. (1977). Recognizing friends by their walk: Gait perception without familiar cues. *Bulletin of the Psychonomic Society, 9,* 353-356.

Fiorentino, M. R. (1973). *Reflex testing methods for evaluating central nervous system development* (2nd ed.). Springfield, Ill: Charles C. Thomas.

Giuliani, C. A. Theories of motor control: New concepts for physical therapy. In *Contemporary management of motor control problems: Proceedings of the II STEP conference* (pp. 29-35). Alexandria, VA: Foundation for Physical Therapy.

Heriza, C. Motor development: Traditional and contemporary theories. In *Contemporary management of motor control problems: Proceedings of the II STEP conference* (pp. 99-126). Alexandria, VA: Foundation for Physical Therapy.

Horak, F., & Nashner, L. (1986). Central programming of postural movements: Adaptations to altered support surface configurations. *Journal of Neurophysiology, 55,* 1369-1381.

Kozlowski, L. T., & Cutting J. E. (1977). Recognizing the sex of a walker from a dynamic point-light display. *Perception and Psychophysics, 21,* 575-580.

Magee, D. J. (1992). *Orthopedic physical assessment* (pp. 352, 376-377). Philadelphia: W. B. Saunders.

Shumway-Cook, A., & Woollacott, M. H. (1995). *Motor control theory and practical applications* (pp. 119-184). Baltimore: Williams & Wilkins.

Vulpe, S. G. (1977). *Vulpe Assessment Battery* (pp. 345-355). Toronto, Ontario: National Institute on Mental Retardation.

Waters, R. L. (1992). Energy expenditure. In J. Perry, *Gait analysis: Normal and pathological function* (pp. 443-459). Thorofare, NJ: SLACK Incorporated.

Wolfson, L., Whipple, R., & Derby, C. A., et al. (1994). Gender differences in the balance of healthy elderly as demonstrated by dynamic posturography. *Journal of Gerontology, 49,* 160-167.

Chapter 7

Batshaw, M. L., & Perret, Y. M. (1981). *Children with handicaps: A medical primer* (pp. 175-176). Baltimore: Paul H. Brookes.

Hunt, G. C. (1990). Examination of lower extremity dysfunction. In J. A. Gould (Ed.), *Orthopaedic and sports physical therapy* (2nd ed., pp. 395-421). St. Louis, MO: C. V. Mosby Co.

Kendall, F. P., McCreary, E. K., & Provance, P. G. (1993). *Muscles testing and function* (4th ed.). Baltimore: Williams & Wilkins.

Klawans, H. L., Goetz, C. G., & Tanner, C. M. (1988). *Common movement disorders.* New York: Raven Press (videotape).

Knutsson, E., & Martensson, A. (1986). Posture and gait in parkinsonian patients. In W. Bles & T. Brandt (Eds.), *Disorders of posture and gait* (pp. 217-252). Amsterdam: Elsevier.

Lower limb orthotics. (1981). New York: New York University Post-Graduate Medical School.

May, B. J. (1996). *Amputations and prosthetics. A case study approach.* Philadelphia: F. A. Davis Co.

Nixon, V. (1985). *Spinal cord injury: A guide to functional outcomes in physical therapy management* (pp. 145-164). Rockville, MD: Aspen Publishers Inc.

Parker, A. W., & Bronks, R. (1980). Gait of children with Down syndrome. *Archives of Physical Medicine and Rehabilitation, 61,* 345-351.

Schmitz, T. J. (1994). Traumatic spinal cord injury. In S. B. O'Sullivan & T. J. Schmitz (Eds.), *Physical rehabilitation: Assessment and treatment* (3rd ed., pp. 533-575). Philadelphia: F. A. Davis Co.

Shurr, D. G., & Cook, T. M. (1990). *Prosthetics and orthotics.* Norwalk, CT: Appleton and Lange.

Singer, S. (1978). *Human genetics: An introduction to the principles of heredity* (2nd ed., pp. 23-28). New York: W. H. Freeman and Co.

Stockiert, B. W. (1995). Peripheral neuropathies. In D. A. Umphred (Ed.), *Neurological rehabilitation* (3rd ed., pp. 360-374). St. Louis, MO: Mosby-Year Book Inc.

Sutherland, D. H. (1984). *Gait disorders in childhood and adolescence.* Baltimore: Williams & Wilkins.

Sutherland, D. H., Olshan, R. A., Biden, E. N., & Wyatt, M. P. (1988). *The development of mature walking.* London: MacKeith Press.

List of Abbreviations

AC	acceleration
AFO	ankle-foot orthosis
AK	above the knee
BOS	base of support
cm	centimeter
COG	center of gravity
COP	center of pressure
DC	deceleration
EA	effort arm
EMG	electromyograph(y)
FF	foot flat
ft	foot
GC	gait cycle
GRFV	ground reaction force vector
HAT	head, arms, and torso
HAV	hallux abductovalgus
HO	heel off
HS	heel strike
IC	initial contact
in	inch
ISw	initial swing
ITB	iliotibial band
LR	loading response
m	meter
mm	millimeter
MMT	manual muscle test
MSt	midstance
MSw	midswing
PSw	preswing
RA	resistance arm
RLA	Rancho Los Amigos
ROM	range of motion
SACH	solid ankle cushion heel
sec	second
STJ	subtalar joint
TO	toe off
TSt	terminal stance
TSw	terminal swing
VO_2	volume of oxygen

Index

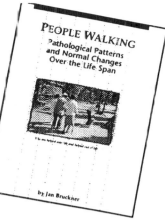